Peter Baker is director of the Men's Health Forum, a leading organization promoting men's health. He was health editor of *Maxim* magazine for four years, and is co-author of *The MANual: The Complete Man's Guide to Life* (1996). He was also the launch editor of www.malehealth.co.uk, the first comprehensive, dedicated men's health website.

'What your doctor would tell you if they had the time. Prevention is better than cure—here's a book that will make you feel better permanently. Recommended.'

Phillip Hodson, psychotherapist and broadcaster

for

Jo, Saskia and Jonah

REAL HEALTH FOR MEN

Peter Baker

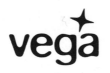

A catalogue record for this book is available
from the British Library.

ISBN 1-84333-014-8

Printed in Great Britain
by Creative Print and Design Wales, Ebbw Vale

© Vega 2002

A member of the Chrysalis Group plc

First published in 2002 by
Vega
64 Brewery Road
London
N7 9NT

Visit our website at www.chrysalisbooks.co.uk

CONTENTS

ACKNOWLEDGEMENTS

Many people have helped me write this book. I owe a particular debt to Dr. Mick Cooper, senior lecturer in counseling at the University of Brighton. Mick commented on drafts too numerous to mention, and was a loyal and supportive friend throughout. Dr. Ian Banks, President of the Men's Health Forum, has also been an inspirational friend and colleague. Special thanks are due to David Plummer, director of the Personal Training Centre, London, for his extensive help with Chapter 4. I would also like to thank Simon Blake, development officer at the Family Planning Association; Mr. Chris Dawson, consultant urologist at the Edith Cavell Hospital, Peterborough; Trefor Lloyd, director of Working With Men; Alan Riley, professor of sexual medicine at the Lancashire Postgraduate School of Medicine and Health, University of Central Lancashire; Nadeem Shafi, health promotion specialist for Southampton Health Promotion Services; Amanda Ursell, a registered nutritionist, state-registered dietitian, and writer and broadcaster on nutrition issues; Dr. Tim Watkin-Jones, a GP with a special interest in men's health; and Dickon Weir-Hughes, chief nurse and director of patient services at the Royal Marsden NHS Trust, London and Surrey. All of the above generously gave their time and expertise to read and comment on various drafts. Finally, I would like to thank my agent, Mandy Little, for her persistence and encouragement at every stage of the development of this book. Needless to say, the contents of this book are solely my responsibility.

The table on pages 136–8 is based on information in M. A. Miller and R. H. Rahe, 'Life-changes scaling for the 1990s,' *Journal of Psychosomatic Research*, 1997, 43(3); pp. 279–92, and is printed with permission.

This book uses both imperial and metric measurements. If necessary, they can be converted as follows:

1 inch = 25.4 millimeters (mm) = 2.54 centimeters (cm)
1 foot = 30.48 centimeters
1 mile = 1.6 kilometers
1 millimeter = 0.039 inches
1 centimeter = 0.39 inches
1 meter (m) = 39 inches
1 kilometer = 0.6 miles
1 ounce (oz) = 28 grams (g)
1 pound (lb) = 0.45 kilograms (kg)
1 stone (st) = 14 pounds = 6.3 kilograms
100 grams = 3.5 ounces
1 kilogram = 2.2 pounds
1 pint = 570 milliliters (ml) = 0.57 liters
1 liter = 1.75 pints

The information in this book is intended for reference only and should not be used in place of advice from a qualified healthcare practitioner. If you have any concerns about your health, you should seek appropriate help.

FOREWORD

I met Peter Baker in 1996 while he was health editor for *Maxim* magazine. Those were the days when men's health as an issue attracted as much media interest as poodle parlors. Journalists reporting on anything male were thin on the ground when it came to taking a serious look at why men die on average six years earlier than women, are four times more likely to take their own lives, have a worse prognosis for just about every disease common to both sexes, yet paradoxically see their doctor half as frequently and often too late. Over the next few years the whole area of men's health was to move to center stage, with politicians falling over themselves to promote research into such hitherto neglected areas as prostate cancer, of which there are an estimated 400,000 new cases a year. This dramatic advance owes itself in no small part to Peter Baker's efforts to provide reliable information in a readable form. His articles in leading magazines and newspapers have been fundamental in breaking the conspiracy of silence surrounding the issue of men's health. An abundance of books on the subject now adorns the booksellers' shelves, ranging from turgid, jargon-ridden tomes perpetuating male myths to superbly referenced, evidence-based, readable masterpieces. Peter Baker not only influenced and stimulated the quality of the best, he has with this book provided the definitive version. Men's health will never be the same again—we hope.

Dr. Ian Banks
President, the Men's Health Forum

REAL WHAT?

How do you feel right now? In great shape, full of energy and positive? Or out of condition, tired and downbeat? If you believe your body and your mind are performing less than optimally, then you've definitely picked up the right book. *Real Health for Men* doesn't promise magic or instant solutions, but it is packed with tried-and-tested information and tips that can stop you feeling as if you're running on empty and start feeling as if you're physically and mentally thriving. This is 21st-century Man's essential guide to complete health.

Whether you're in need of fine tuning or a complete overhaul, this book will show how you can feel better now. If it's more energy you're after, you'll find out how to make simple changes to your physical-activity levels, diet or sleeping habits that will make a big difference. If you're feeling stressed out, you'll discover easy ways to relax and organize your time better. If you're having sexual problems, perhaps with maintaining an erection or because you are ejaculating too quickly, you'll learn about treatments and techniques that can lead to a near-immediate improvement. And if you're ill, you'll understand how to get yourself better as quickly as possible.

Many men believe the future offers only baldness, an ever-growing belly, a sex life that flops after 40 and a heart attack at 55. While it's unfortunately true that whatever happens to your hair is largely down to genetics, you certainly don't have to settle for a steady slide toward senility. However old you are, making a few key changes now will radically increase your chances of feeling good about yourself, keeping fit, enjoying an active sex life and avoiding heart disease and cancer, the two biggest threats to men's health. In short, you can live a much longer—and happier—life.

Real Health for Men aims to be practical, not weird and wacky. You won't be told that the secret of good health lies in developing a six-pack stomach, let alone weekly colonic irrigation or a diet of lentils, rice cakes and a hundred different types of seaweed. It does include information about some so-called complementary treatments—such as acupuncture and herbalism—but only when there's solid evidence to back them up. The overall aim of the book is not to turn men into health freaks—the kind of guys who are obsessed with checking their blood pressure as well as the fat content of every turnip they eat—but rather to make keeping healthy seem as ordinary, and as important, as enjoying a beer with friends after work.

This book is a manual, not a novel, so you don't have to read it from beginning to end to find it helpful. You'll pick up tons of useful information by simply dipping in and out of the sections that interest you when you're commuting to work or bored with television soaps. Think of it like a car handbook: if you've got a problem with your exhaust you probably won't want to read about spark plugs or how to fix the windscreen wipers, unless you happen to be fascinated by every aspect of vehicle maintenance. So, if you're mainly interested in giving up smoking or improving your physical fitness you don't have to wade through pages of information about testicle problems or tackling depression.

It may be, of course, that once you've finished the sections that most concern you, you'll be curious to find out more, either straightaway or maybe even in six months' or a year's time. While the book is designed to be read in individual sections, it also fits together as a whole to provide a comprehensive guide to improving your health as a man. If you do have the time, the energy and the motivation to work through the entire book—and to implement its many suggestions—there's little doubt that you'll be well on your way to becoming Mr. Healthy, both physically and mentally.

You've certainly picked a good time to get interested in your health. Just 20 years ago, the majority of men felt about as motivated to improve their health as they did to prepare the evening meal or clean the lavatory. Men may still be reluctant to pick up a toilet brush, but there can be no doubt that ever-increasing numbers are now keen to improve their health. It's definitely no longer taboo for a man to take better care of himself, a fact clearly reflected in the sales of men's health and fitness magazines and the growing numbers of men taking time out to work out.

Finally, it's important to realize that no book should be used to diagnose and treat any potentially serious illness. If you have any worries about your health, or any unusual or unexplained symptoms, your best bet is to see a healthcare professional as soon as possible. One of the most important messages of this book is that men don't have to wait until they've developed a lump the size of a basketball or a pain worse than a Mike Tyson punch below the belt before they seek medical help. Seeing a doctor isn't a waste of time, it isn't something to be embarrassed about, and it certainly isn't a sign of weakness. In fact, you're entitled to—and deserve—nothing less than the best possible healthcare from the medical profession and, even more importantly, from yourself.

CHAPTER 1

FROM LIVING HELL TO LIVING WELL:

THE MEN'S HEALTH CHALLENGE

Many scientists now believe that most humans are, in theory at least, able to live for 115 or even 120 years. Since the life expectancy of most men in the Western world today is around 70–75, it's clear that too many of us are expiring well before we need to. Although the next generation of men will undoubtedly benefit from many new medical breakthroughs, if we want to enjoy longer, healthier lives there's no need to sit around waiting for scientists to come up with a cure for cancer or a new kind of margarine that prevents heart attacks. Simply making a few changes to our diet, becoming more physically active and quitting smoking could be enough to make a massive difference. Finding better ways of coping with stress, paying more attention to our sexual health and seeing a doctor when we feel unwell would also help hugely. So what's stopping us?

Health isn't a 'man thing'

Although men's attitudes are now beginning to change, too many men have for too long believed that being interested in health is about as manly and desirable as spending their evenings darning socks or flower-arranging. It's not what 'normal' men do—health is for women and children or wimpish hypochondriacs who spend their time wandering around terrified they're having a heart attack or developing a brain tumor. 'Real' men are supposed to be tough and always in control; being ill is unmanly because it can make us feel weak, vulnerable, and dependent on others. Can you imagine a guy like Russell Crowe, the muscular Maximus in the film

Gladiator, tucked up in bed with a cold flannel on his forehead and a nurse emptying his bedpan? Let's face it, Arnold Schwarzenegger is as likely to have a baby.

Many men are about as keen to seek medical help as to be hit in the groin by a fiercely struck football. In fact, they'll probably put it off until they've developed a raging fever and are covered in more red spots than there are craters on the moon. It's not just that men hate asking for help or don't want to look stupid when the doctor tells them they haven't got the life-threatening illness they've spent the last five nights lying awake worrying about. For some, it's also because they've convinced themselves that every trip to the clinic inevitably involves a humiliating encounter between a doctor and their genitals. Perhaps this absurd fantasy is understandable, though, given that many young men's first medical examination involved a testicle-grabbing school nurse whose communication skills consisted of little more than saying 'cough'.

The risks men take

'Real' men also take risks. In fact, risk-taking behaviors is one important way in which males of all ages prove their masculinity to themselves and each other. Afraid of appearing timid, boys play 'chicken' on railway tracks and young men joy-ride fast cars through the streets. Adult men enjoy dangerous sports—skydiving, hang-gliding or mountain-climbing—while many more smoke, drink too much or practice unsafe sex. In the workplace, too, men are likely to lift weights that are too heavy for them or walk around a construction site without a hard hat. It seems a man's still gotta do what he's gotta do, regardless of the consequences for his health.

Men's attitudes toward their health don't seem quite so strange when we consider the role models they've been brought up to emulate. After all, it's hard to imagine Rambo checking his testicles for lumps or Captain Kirk worrying about eating enough fresh fruit and vegetables. Super-heroes are not likely to call off their mission to safeguard humanity because the work's a bit stressful or because they might end up with a few bruises (or much worse). For these guys, good physical and mental health is a low, if not non-existent, priority and, like them, real-life men tend to view their bodies as virtually indestructible, Robocop-like machines.

Ignorance isn't bliss

Not being interested in health also means that men are often very ignorant about it. Too many of us believe—wrongly—that simply being physically fit is enough to guarantee good health. A *Reader's Digest* survey found that just 11 per cent of men could correctly identify the position of the prostate gland on a diagram of a male

WHAT DO MEN DIE OF?

HEART DISEASE. The world's biggest single cause of death—and the main cause of premature death. Almost 640,000 men a year are killed by the disease in the UK, USA, Canada, and Australia alone; in those countries, it accounts for 39 per cent of all male deaths. Men are much more likely than women to die prematurely from heart disease: the death rates for men aged 35–74 are up to three times those for women.

CANCER. The second biggest cause of death; world-wide, almost four million men die from cancer each year. The biggest killers are, in descending order, cancer of the lung, stomach, bowel, prostate, mouth/pharynx, liver, esophagus and bladder. In the UK, USA, Canada, and Australia, there are one-and-a-half times as many male as female deaths from all the main cancers that affect both sexes.

ACCIDENTS. A major cause of premature death among men. More than 75,400 men a year die in accidents in the UK, USA, Canada, and Australia; of these deaths, almost half are caused by traffic accidents. Men are about twice as likely as women to die in an accident, and about 90 per cent of all serious injuries at work affect men.

SUICIDE. More than 33,000 men take their own lives each year in the UK, USA, Canada, and Australia. Men die by suicide in far greater numbers than women: in these countries, the ratio of male to female deaths is 4:1.

HOMICIDE. More than 20,000 men a year are killed by other people—overwhelmingly other men—in the UK, USA, Canada, and Australia. A man is over three-and-a-half times more likely to be a victim of a homicide than a woman.

AIDS. This has emerged as a major cause of premature death for men in the past 20 years: some six million have died throughout the world since the beginning of the epidemic in the early 1980s. Well over 600,000 men in North America, Western Europe and Australia have developed AIDS, and, in these countries, men make up over 80 per cent of all reported cases.

THE RISKS MEN TAKE

Who's more likely to:

Smoke	Men
Drink at dangerous levels	Men
Drink and drive	Men
Use illegal drugs (cannabis, ecstasy, cocaine, etc.)	Men
Eat unhealthy food	Men
Be overweight	Men
Practice unsafe sex	Men
Play dangerous sports	Men
Avoid the doctor	Men
Avoid the dentist	Men

body (ironically, women were better informed about this than men—16 per cent got it right). Even more worryingly, almost 50 per cent of men admitted they knew nothing at all about either prostate or testicular cancer. Another survey found that just one-third of men aged 25–34 knew how to examine themselves for signs of testicular cancer.

Men don't have periods—or babies

Men lack an obvious biological mechanism that regularly makes them feel aware of, and in touch with, their bodies. Although there is evidence of a natural testosterone cycle, it isn't significant enough for men to notice and can't be compared with the much more perceptible rhythms of a woman's monthly menstrual cycle. You don't need to be a gynecologist to realize that men can't get pregnant, either, and they don't experience a rapid, powerful hormonal change equivalent to the female menopause. What's more, men's reproductive systems don't require them to maintain any regular contact with healthcare services. Men don't need to see a healthcare professional about their contraception—they can buy condoms from a supermarket or pharmacy—whereas virtually all forms of women's contraception must be prescribed. Although men can be affected emotionally and physically by a partner's pregnancy, it's highly unlikely they will feel the need to seek medical attention. They certainly won't be having their blood, urine, blood pressure, and belly size regularly monitored in the months leading up to the birth of their child.

Do the medics care?

The medical profession has so far done little to encourage men to use its services. Most clinics are open during normal working hours only, restricting access for men who work full-time, and there are very few services specializing in men's health problems. Even if a man does visit his doctor, the odds are that the consultation will be less than satisfactory: many men find it hard to talk about their health worries, so unless they see someone who understands their reticence, they may never get around to saying what's really on their mind. There is evidence to suggest that some healthcare professionals also assume that men are less likely to be seriously ill, especially with a mental-health problem.

Doctors can be seriously under-informed about men's problems. Even though one in 10 men is affected by erectile dysfunction (impotence), a survey by the UK Impotence Association found that nearly half of those men who went to their doctor found him or her unhelpful. Indeed, for almost a quarter of patients, the doctor took no action at all.

Finally, research into male-specific health problems isn't yet seen as a priority. This is exemplified by the case of prostate cancer. It's a potentially deadly and increasingly common disease, but astonishingly little is yet known about its causes or the most effective treatments. There can be few other areas of healthcare where men have been so badly let down by the medical system.

MEN AND WOMEN: WHO'S HEALTHIER?

Women certainly live longer. The average woman currently lives about five to eight years longer than the average man, and she's nine times more likely to reach the age of 100. In fact, men are more likely to die at any age, with particularly sharp differences in death rates between the ages of 15 and 35. Incredibly, males start dying faster than females even before they're born: although at least 115 males are conceived for every 100 females, just 105 boys are born for every 100 girls because of a much higher rate of miscarriages and stillbirths of male fetuses. The evidence about whether men or women suffer worse levels of ill-health before they die isn't as clear-cut, however. The statistics suggest that women tend to have more experience of illness than men but that their illnesses tend to be less serious; in other words, women are sicker in the short-run while men are sicker in the long-run.

THINGS YOU DIDN'T KNOW ABOUT WHY MEN DIE SOONER THAN WOMEN

○ Men's natural body shape could put them at greater risk of dying sooner than women. When women put on weight, it tends to be spread around their body. When men put on weight, it's usually concentrated around their waists. This matters, because having a beer belly creates a much higher risk of 'furred up' arteries and heart disease—fat stored here is very mobile and is quickly released into the bloodstream in response to stimuli such as stress.

○ The blood women lose during their monthly periods reduces their iron levels and may therefore help to prevent hardening of the arteries and cut their heart-attack risk. Men obviously don't lose blood in the same way, but research suggests that donating blood might be an effective substitute. Male blood donors aged 42–60 run just 12 per cent of the heart-attack risk of non-blood donors, according to a study of almost 3000 Finnish men.

○ The male sex hormone testosterone may increase the level of low-density lipoproteins (LDL), the 'bad' type of cholesterol that increases the risk of heart disease, and may also reduce the level of high-density lipoproteins (HDL), the 'good' type of cholesterol that protects against heart disease. But the impact of testosterone is much less than that of the female sex hormone estrogen. This helps keep women's LDL cholesterol levels low and is also an 'antioxidant'. This means it can help neutralize 'free radicals', nasty molecules created naturally during normal metabolic processes (as well as by a range of pollutants), which whizz around the body damaging cells and blood vessels. That's why women start to be at much greater risk of heart disease when their estrogen levels fall after the menopause.

○ Men's greater vulnerability to health problems could be related to their chromosomal make-up. Some scientists believe that because a female has two 'X' chromosomes, an abnormal gene on one of them can be compensated for by a normal gene on the other. A male, on the other hand, has one X chromosome and one Y chromosome, and so cannot rely on an alternative chromosome if a gene on his single X or single Y chromosome is defective.

○ There's increasing evidence that having an intimate relationship with a partner, as well as a rich and diverse network of social relationships, protects people against ill-health and contributes to a reduced risk of death. Women tend to enjoy more—and closer—relationships than men, possibly giving them an important health advantage.

The upshot

Although being born with male genes and hormones may slightly increase the chances of dying prematurely, any reasonably skilled poker player will tell you that being dealt less favorable cards doesn't mean that the game is inevitably lost. We all have the ability to make the most of our genetic and biological potential and to improve significantly our health and well-being. The biggest problem we face as men is not our biology but the way in which we've been brought up to think about our health—that is, as little as possible.

But men are now starting to take their health more seriously. They are generally under much less pressure to conform to the 'real man' stereotype and far fewer regard taking better care of themselves as 'sissy stuff'. This makes it much easier for men to accept that they might not be indestructible after all, to give up at least some of their risk-taking behaviorss, and even to admit that they might sometimes have a health problem.

In the last few years, some well-known men have 'come out' about their prostate cancer, including Senator Bob Dole and General Norman Schwarzkopf in the US, and Nelson Mandela in South Africa. The American baseball player John Kruk and the British jockey Bob Champion have spoken publicly about their experience of testicular cancer. The British Olympic rower Steve Redgrave has also been open about his diabetes and colitis. These public figures have made it easier for others to feel more comfortable about seeking help if they spot the symptoms of these diseases. The advent of Viagra, the first oral treatment for erectile dysfunction (impotence), has had an even bigger effect. Increasing numbers of men are now willing to consult their doctors about what used to be considered the most private of health problems.

There's more help available for any man who decides to take action to improve his health. As well as magazines and books, there are Internet sites and a small but growing number of doctors and clinics now taking a special interest in men's health. Men are starting to organize self-help groups and campaigns to push for more services and research into conditions like testicular and prostate cancers. Some governments, even, are showing the first signs of taking men's health more seriously; they've realized they can't improve the overall health of their nations unless they begin to do so.

There's still some way to go before most of us can expect to live to 100, but it's completely realistic for many more of us to live well into our 80s and 90s. What's more, making the changes that will enable us to live longer will make us feel a whole lot better now—we certainly won't have to wait 30, 40, or even 50 years to begin to see the pay-offs. Want to get going? Then read on.

CHAPTER 2

ARE YOU MR. HEALTHY?

Y ou probably don't think twice about giving your car an annual service. You may even check your computer for viruses or give the dog an occasional once-over for fleas. But what about *your* body? How often do you monitor the state of your own health? This chapter enables you to work out your own 'Health Profile' in the comfort of your living room—and without a doctor in sight.

You might be surprised to see that the Health Profile refers to issues like having a good laugh, feeling loved, or being part of a community. But they're included for a very good reason: there's increasing evidence that factors like the quality of our relationships with others, how we deal with stress, and even how much control we have over our work can have an enormous impact on our physical health. It's no longer credible to blame ill-health simply on bad luck (such as family inheritance), bacteria or viruses, exposure to toxic chemicals (whether tobacco smoke or asbestos), accidents, or the long-term effects of a poor diet.

The Health Profile, then, covers much more than physical health. Like the rest of this book, it takes a much wider view of what constitutes genuine health and well-being. That's because it's perfectly possible to have a body that's in A1 condition and still be unhealthy. How so? Since a man's mental state forms a central part of his overall well-being, someone who's depressed, continually anxious, has panic attacks, or is a compulsive gambler or a workaholic cannot be said to be truly healthy. Good mental or emotional health is as important an objective as good physical health.

This chapter enables you to assess the state of the key components of your physical and mental well-being. On the following pages you'll find over 60 statements, each relating to a different aspect of your health. All you have to do is note whether you agree or disagree with each of them, and tick each box you agree with. Take your time and be as honest with yourself as possible—the point isn't to look good but to find out for yourself how healthy you really are.

SECTION 1. LIFESTYLE.

☐ I eat fresh fruit and vegetables every day.
☐ I limit the amount of fat I eat.
☐ On average, I drink no more than one or two alcoholic drinks a day.
☐ I'm physically active (e.g. brisk walking) for a total of at least 30 minutes a day, five days a week or I exercise vigorously (e.g. running or fast cycling) for at least 20 minutes, three times a week.
☐ I never smoke.
☐ My waist circumference is below 37 inches.
☐ I get all the sleep I need.
☐ I avoid the sun or use a sunscreen.

SECTION 2. EMOTIONAL HEALTH.

☐ I feel good about myself.
☐ I like the way I look.
☐ I mostly feel optimistic about the future.
☐ I cope well with stress.
☐ I value feeling 'negative' emotions (e.g. sadness or guilt) as well as 'positive' emotions (e.g. joy or excitement).
☐ I find it easy to talk about or show my feelings.
☐ I regularly have a good laugh.
☐ I feel comfortable about telling other people what I want.

SECTION 3. WORK.

☐ I have regular work.
☐ I'm satisfied with my working life.
☐ My work doesn't expose me to any significant health and safety risks (e.g. radiation, toxic chemicals, noise, repetitive strain injury).
☐ My work is largely free of unpleasant stress.
☐ I have enough control over how I do my job.
☐ I've achieved a good balance between my home life and my working life.
☐ I work 40 or fewer hours a week (unless I choose to work for longer).
☐ I take at least 20 days' holiday leave each year.

SECTION 4. RELATIONSHIPS.

- ❏ I have a supportive social network of family and/or friends.
- ❏ I feel part of a community.
- ❏ I enjoy a good relationship with a partner.
- ❏ I feel loved.
- ❏ I regularly touch (e.g. hug, cuddle, kiss) the people I'm close to.
- ❏ I can listen to other people without interrupting them.
- ❏ If my relationship with a partner was in serious trouble, I'd consider going to couples counseling.
- ❏ I often feel a sense of connection to the natural world and/or a spiritual feeling of interconnectedness.

SECTION 5. SEXUAL HEALTH.

- ❏ If I started a new sexual relationship, I'd practice safer sex (e.g. using a condom during intercourse; note that the term 'safer' is used rather than 'safe': condoms do not totally rule out the risks either of unwanted pregnancy or sexually transmitted infections).
- ❏ If I was about to start a new sexual relationship, I'd seriously consider having a check-up for sexually transmitted infections (e.g. gonorrhea and chlamydia).
- ❏ If I developed a sexual problem, such as erectile dysfunction (impotence) or premature ejaculation, I'd consult a health professional.
- ❏ I masturbate if I feel the need to do so without feeling any guilt or shame.
- ❏ I believe I still have a lot to learn about lovemaking.
- ❏ I feel confident enough to tell my partner what I want during sex.
- ❏ I feel sexually satisfied.
- ❏ I'm comfortable with my sexual identity (e.g. straight, gay, or bisexual).

SECTION 6. COPING WITH ILL-HEALTH.

- ❏ I believe there's more to recovering from ill-health than relying on drugs or surgery.
- ❏ I find it easy to rest if it's a necessary part of recovering from an illness.
- ❏ I wouldn't hesitate to consult a health professional if I was unwell (except for minor problems like colds or flu).
- ❏ I'd seriously consider trying a complementary therapy (e.g. osteopathy, acupuncture, homeopathy) if I was unwell, especially if mainstream medicine couldn't help.

❑ If I was unwell, I'd feel comfortable about asking for help from other people, such as friends and family.

❑ If I had a major health problem, I'd consider going to a support group to talk to other people in the same position.

❑ If I felt depressed, or was worried about my emotional health, I'd consider seeing a counselor or therapist.

❑ If I wasn't satisfied with any medical advice I'd been given, I'd ask for a second opinion.

SECTION 7. PREVENTING ILL-HEALTH.

❑ I'm registered with a doctor.

❑ I have my blood pressure checked at least once every three years.

❑ I have my urine checked for diabetes or a kidney infection at least once every three years.

❑ I have my cholesterol level checked at least once every three years (or, if you're under 30, you intend to have it tested after that age).

❑ I regularly check my whole body for signs of unusual bleeding, sores or discharge, lumps, swellings, or changes in mole size or color.

❑ I see a dentist for a check-up at least once a year.

❑ I have my eyes checked at least once every two years (whether or not I wear glasses or contact lenses).

❑ I'd welcome the opportunity to have a complete health check-up by a health professional at least once every three years.

SECTION 8. HEALTH PROBLEMS.

❑ I generally feel well and have plenty of energy.

❑ I don't suffer from chronic aches and pains (e.g. back pain).

❑ I recover quickly from injuries or illness.

❑ I'm neither gaining nor losing weight rapidly.

❑ I rarely feel depressed or anxious.

❑ I almost always achieve a good enough erection for sex.

❑ I have no problems with urination (e.g. an interrupted or weak flow, dribbling, pain, or a need to go to the toilet several times during the night).

❑ I have no unusual or unexplained physical symptoms (e.g. chest pains, lumps, changes in bowel habits, a persistent cough or sore throat, unusual bleeding or discharge, problems swallowing).

Your Health Profile

For each statement you agreed with, award yourself 1 point. For each statement you disagreed with, award yourself 0 points. Add up the total number of points you've scored in each section, and use the tables below to get a sense of your health strengths and weaknesses.

SECTION 1. LIFESTYLE.

Your health isn't simply determined by your genes, whether you happen to be exposed to any nasty bugs, the signs of the zodiac, or any sins you may have committed in a past life. You may well love your pizzas and Pilsners but there's no avoiding the fact that too many of any of them could mean you'll end up in your local hospital's cardiac unit.

SCORE	ANALYSIS
0–4	Your lifestyle could be putting your health at risk. You could be poorly informed about what's healthy and what isn't, or you are unwilling or unable to change your behavior. You're probably willing to take risks with your health.
5–6	You're doing well in most areas but you're still missing some of the essential building blocks of optimum health.
7–8	You're either lying or you're already aged 108! Alternatively, you could simply be very health conscious, in which case you are much less likely to be affected by a wide range of lifestyle-related illnesses (such as heart disease, cancer, and diabetes).

SECTION 2. EMOTIONAL HEALTH.

It's easy to believe that your emotional life and your physical health are completely separate. But scientists have proved that, regardless of whether you smoke, drink too much, or spend all day slumped on the sofa watching *South Park* videos, feeling stressed, anxious, or depressed can increase your risk of catching a cold or developing heart disease. Your emotional life matters for its own sake, too—after all, do you really want to spend your life feeling miserable?

SCORE	ANALYSIS
0–4	Your emotional life needs an overhaul. You could well be suffering from low self-esteem, stress, anxiety, and even depression. You may struggle to cope with difficult life-events and find it hard to understand, communicate, or control your feelings.
5–6	Your emotional life is generally robust but is not without its weak areas. You are probably mostly positive and optimistic but you may well also experience difficult periods of anxiety, hopelessness, and self-doubt.
7–8	You are almost certainly emotionally healthy with a positive sense of yourself and the world. Your high levels of self-esteem, self-confidence, and optimism should contribute to good all-round health.

SECTION 3. WORK.

Even if you don't work down a coal mine or at a nuclear power plant, your work can still affect your health. If health and safety procedures are ignored, if the job is stressful, if you can't control your workload or working hours, then you could still be heading for trouble. Having almost any kind of regular job, though, provides a sense of status and purpose, while being unemployed can prove demoralizing and depressing.

SCORE	ANALYSIS
0–4	Your working life could cause you health problems, whether as a result of an unhealthy or unsafe environment, stress, or long working hours. Being unemployed is also a health risk factor.
5–6	Work is not all it could be. In many respects it's going well, but stress or poor working conditions could eventually affect your health.

SCORE	ANALYSIS
7–8	Your working life seems essentially safe, healthy, and stimulating. You probably have a high level of work satisfaction and a good balance between work and the rest of your life.

SECTION 4. RELATIONSHIPS.

Relationships are about much more than sex and having someone to go to the movies with on Saturday nights (crucial though these two things are for most of us). Believe it or not, the richness of your social networks, as well as the quality of your most intimate relationships, can have a huge impact on your health and well-being. If you feel loved and supported then it is much more likely that you will enjoy good health than if you feel isolated and lonely.

SCORE	ANALYSIS
0–4	You might well often feel lonely and disconnected from other people. This is a health risk in itself; it can also affect how quickly you seek help for a health problem and could delay your recovery.
5–6	You probably have some good relationships but also feel as if this part of your life is under-developed; you may not feel as close to the people you value as you would like.
7–8	You generally feel well-connected and close to other people and perhaps to the wider natural and/or spiritual world, too. This could help protect you against ill-health.

SECTION 5. SEXUAL HEALTH.

Sex five times a night, a different partner twice a week, and a penis that's 10 inches long—these 'achievements' have nothing to do with good sexual health. Sexual health is actually about feeling comfortable with your sexuality and enjoying your sexual experiences, as well as avoiding or promptly treating sexually transmitted infections and other sexual problems like erectile dysfunction (impotence).

SCORE	ANALYSIS
0–4	Your sex life could well be in need of a serious overhaul. Your health, as well as that of your partners, could be at risk, too, from your sexual behavior. You may also have feelings of confusion, embarrassment, or even shame about your sexuality which could prevent you from seeking help for sexual problems and cause you stress and anxiety.
5–6	Your sex life has many positive aspects but is not as healthy as it could be. It may be that you need to pay more attention to practicing safer sex, or to increasing your sexual satisfaction or resolving doubts about your sexual identity.
7–8	You're sexually responsible, have few hang-ups and enjoy yourself in bed (or wherever else you choose to have sex).

SECTION 6. COPING WITH ILL-HEALTH.

On finding out they're ill, some men react by heading straight for the gym or a five-mile run. They believe that health problems can somehow be 'sweated out' or that, so long as they're still physically fit, there can't really be anything seriously wrong with them. But they might be better advised to walk slowly to the doctor's to find out exactly what's wrong. It can also be helpful to accept that there's often a role for the less scientific but more user-friendly complementary therapies.

SCORE	ANALYSIS
0–4	You're not very good at dealing with illness, perhaps because you don't like feeling weak, vulnerable, or dependent. You probably see health problems as some sort of mechanical defect of a particular body part rather than in the context of your overall well-being.

SCORE	ANALYSIS
5–6	You're reasonably good at coping with ill-health, although you're less likely to believe that there are effective treatments beyond the scope of the drugs or surgery offered by mainstream medicine.
7–8	You're a model patient. You don't hesitate to seek the most appropriate help for your problem, you're comfortable about appearing vulnerable and dependent, and you accept that there's a close connection between your mind and body.

SECTION 7. PREVENTING ILL-HEALTH.

When you travel on an airplane, you expect the ground crew and pilots to have thoroughly checked every part of the plane before it takes off. You'd certainly prefer that to an accident followed by an investigation into what might have gone wrong. But do you follow the same principle when it comes to your health? Do you regularly get yourself checked out so you can head off serious problems well before they arise? If you want to avoid a crash landing in the local hospital, it's certainly worth making the time for a few simple preventive health checks.

SCORE	ANALYSIS
0–4	You may well pay little attention to your health, so you're less likely to detect the first signs of any health problems and more likely to delay seeking help.
5–6	You can see the value of some preventive health checks but aren't yet consistent in your approach. Some problems could become more serious before you discover them.
7–8	You accept the value of preventive health checks and believe healthcare professionals can help you. You're more likely to spot potential health problems and seek help quickly if you do.

SECTION 8. HEALTH PROBLEMS.

You don't need to be a brain surgeon to realize that the sooner symptoms are detected and diagnosed, the easier it is to treat and cure them. Men who delay going into hospital when they have a heart attack are much more likely to die, and testicular cancer, for example, can now almost always be cured so long as it's treated immediately after a lump's been discovered. Simply hoping that a problem will go away or somehow cure itself, or that it's bound to be something trivial, doesn't constitute a rational or viable survival strategy.

SCORE	ANALYSIS
0–7	If you haven't already done so, get medical advice. Your problems could well be caused by relatively minor illnesses—or might be signs of something rather more serious. Whatever the cause, there's no good reason why you should have to live with discomfort or pain.
8	You appear to be in good health. This isn't a complete list of symptoms, however, so if you have any other problems that are worrying you, or causing any discomfort, make an appointment to see your doctor.

What now?

Don't worry if you haven't scored top marks in every—or any—of the sections. Very few people will do so, especially if they've been totally honest. And there's no need to panic if you've recorded low scores in some—or even all—of the sections. Rather than feeling daunted or disheartened by what you've learnt about yourself, see the changes you need to make as a challenge and an opportunity. It might help to think of yourself as an athlete in training. If you didn't have a coach who ruthlessly dissected and criticized your technique, you'd never know what specific problems had to be tackled in order to improve your overall performance. Even if you've always come last in every race, with the right help and support you will almost certainly begin to increase your speed and strength. Whether you're preparing for the Olympics, or simply want to boost your health, it's never too late to start getting into better shape.

CHAPTER 3

THE AGES OF MAN

How do you feel about getting older? If you're in your teens, you probably can't wait to be seen as an adult. You'll then be able to take greater control of your life, buy alcohol and cigarettes legally—if that's what you really want—and, with luck, have lots of sex (with other people, that is, rather than yourself). If you've reached 20, you're pretty much at your physical peak and you're probably worrying less about ageing than the prospect of the earth being invaded by aliens. If you're 35, however, there's a good chance you'd like to start slowing down your biological clock. You could well be spending more time peering anxiously at your steadily-expanding waistline—you might even start saying 'no' to that fourth slice of deep-pan pizza—and wondering whether you should join a gym. If you're 50, you probably want the ageing process to stop altogether. You can easily find yourself wondering when you might have to start taking Viagra or even whether it's really worth having cosmetic surgery to remove those wrinkles. And if you're now 70, you may well have already resigned yourself to what could seem like an inevitable and headlong plummet toward infirmity, senility, and, finally, oblivion.

But ageing doesn't have to be like this. It's undeniable that our bodies will change and that we'll become increasingly vulnerable to a variety of health problems. Yet it's also perfectly possible for us to age well. We can still enjoy life, maintain a sense of humor, be open to new ideas, and accept the past as well as the future. We can ensure an optimal level of physical and mental health by understanding how ageing affects the body, knowing how to reduce the risks of ill-health and learning about the symptoms to watch out for. If we do develop a health problem, moreover, we can also help ourselves by not simply and pessimistically blaming our age—something that can never be reversed—but by finding out about its specific, and probably treatable, causes.

Through the experiences of four typical men, this chapter explores the main changes we face as we age and some of the steps that can be taken to remain healthy at every stage.

Mr. Young—20 years old

YOUR HEALTH ASSETS

- Physically, you're at your prime and your risk of developing a serious physical illness is low.
- Muscle strength is at its height.
- Your metabolism is firing on all cylinders, making it harder to put on weight.
- Testosterone production has almost reached its peak.
- Your immune system has only recently passed its prime.
- You probably enjoy high levels of enthusiasm and energy.

YOUR HEALTH RISKS

- Accidents. This is your biggest risk of injury or death, especially as a result of dangerous driving.
- Anxiety. You could well be plagued with self-doubts about your appearance, sexual relationships, sexual orientation and employment prospects.
- Boozing. You're in the age group most likely to be drinking at unsafe levels and to be binge drinking.
- Drugs. You're in the age group most likely to be using illegal drugs. The long-term, regular use of most drugs causes physical and mental health problems.
- Fast food. You're more likely than older men to satisfy your hunger with high-fat junk food. This could eventually cause problems like weight gain and furred-up arteries.
- Sexual problems. Thirty per cent of men are affected by premature ejaculation and 19 per cent worry about their performance.
- Sexually transmitted infections (STIs). Sexually active men of your age have more partners than older men, creating an increased risk of catching an STI.
- Smoking. You're at the peak age for cigarette smoking.
- Suicide. A major cause of death for men of your age—and the rates are increasing.
- Testicular cancer. You've just entered the highest risk age group for this disease (it's the most common cancer among 20–35 year olds).
- Violence. You're particularly at risk of being attacked and injured by other men.

YOUR HEALTH PRIORITIES

○ Quit smoking.
○ Drink a moderate amount of alcohol. Ideally, this should be no more than a drink or two a day.
○ Exercise regularly.
○ Practice safer sex (i.e. by using a condom during intercourse).
○ Eat plenty of fresh fruit and vegetables and less fat.
○ Drive with care (and always wear a seat belt).
○ Avoid violence.
○ Don't use illegal drugs.
○ Talk to friends, or perhaps a counselor, about any feelings of inadequacy, anxiety, or depression.
○ Remember you're not invulnerable.

YOUR REGULAR HEALTH CHECKS

(for all 20–29-year-olds)
○ Blood pressure (high blood pressure is a risk factor for heart disease): every three years.
○ body-mass (your weight/height ratio): every month (see page 58).
○ Cholesterol (a high level is a risk factor for heart disease): every three years (but only if there's a family history of heart problems).
○ Dental examination: every year.
○ Eye examination: every two years (every year if you wear glasses or contact lenses).
○ HIV: only if you feel you have been at risk and want to know for sure.
○ Sexually transmitted infections (except HIV): if there are symptoms. If not, and you are sexually active and changing partners, consider an annual check.
○ Skin cancer: examine yourself (or ask a friend) every two months for changes in mole size, shape, or color and any other odd-looking skin growths.
○ Testicular cancer: examine yourself once a month (see page 256).
○ Urine analysis (for diabetes or a kidney infection): every three years.

Mr. Thirtysomething—35 years old

YOUR HEALTH ASSETS

- ○ Your age makes it unlikely that you'll suffer from a serious physical health problem.
- ○ You've probably developed the emotional capacity to sustain a long-term intimate relationship.
- ○ You're more likely to see your work as a source of satisfaction than just 'a job'.

YOUR HEALTH RISKS

- ○ Boozing. There's a one in three chance you're drinking excessively.
- ○ HIV. Most men who know they're HIV positive find out by the age of 35.
- ○ Prostatitis. This inflammation of the prostate gland is especially common in the 20–40 age group.
- ○ Sexual problems. One-third of men of this age are affected by premature ejaculation.
- ○ Smoking. You're in the age group of smokers who puff through most cigarettes.
- ○ Stress. You may be finding it hard to balance work and the rest of your life.
- ○ Suicide. You're in the age group with the highest level of suicide.
- ○ Testicular cancer. You're still in the highest risk age group.
- ○ Weight. The mid- to late-30s is a critical period for weight gain in men.

YOUR HEALTH PRIORITIES

- ○ Quit smoking.
- ○ Drink alcohol at safe levels.
- ○ Exercise regularly.
- ○ Practice safer sex (i.e. by using a condom during intercourse).
- ○ Eat plenty of fresh fruit and vegetables and less fat.
- ○ Keep your weight at a safe, healthy level.
- ○ Don't use illegal drugs.
- ○ Tackle stress by keeping your work commitments under control and finding ways to relax.
- ○ Talk to friends, or perhaps a counselor, about feelings of anxiety or depression.

YOUR REGULAR HEALTH CHECKS

(for all 30–44-year-olds)
- Blood pressure (high blood pressure is a risk factor for heart disease): every two years.
- body-mass (your weight/height ratio): every month (see page 58).
- Cholesterol (a high level is a risk factor for heart disease): every three years.
- Dental examination: every year.
- Eye examination: every two years (every year if you wear glasses or contact lenses).
- HIV: only if you feel you have been at risk and want to know for sure.
- Sexually transmitted infections (except HIV): if there are symptoms. If not, and you are sexually active and changing partners, consider an annual check.
- Skin cancer: examine yourself (or ask a friend) every two months for changes in mole size, shape, or color and other odd-looking skin growths.
- Testicular cancer: examine yourself once a month (see page 256).
- Urine analysis (for diabetes or a kidney infection): every two years.

Mr. Mid-life—50 years old

YOUR HEALTH ASSETS

- You've probably abandoned much of the risk-taking behavior of your earlier years (e.g. fast driving, excessive drinking).
- You're likely to have developed a network of significant relationships.
- Your chances of developing testicular cancer are now dramatically reduced.
- Basic lifestyle changes—exercising more, eating better, stopping smoking—can still make a huge difference to your health.

YOUR HEALTH RISKS

- Cancer. Although you're still well below the peak age for most cancers, you should nonetheless be particularly alert for the symptoms of cancers of the bladder, bowel, prostate, and skin (see page 226).
- Depression. You could be affected by the 'mid-life crisis' (see page 125).
- Diabetes. The risk of developing diabetes increases after the age of 40. The symptoms include thirst, producing more urine than usual, and fatigue.
- Heart disease. Your risk of heart problems has now increased substantially,

although you're not yet in the highest-risk age group.
- ○ Hernia. This is much more common in men aged 50 plus.
- ○ Sexual problems. Almost one fifth of men in their 50s experience erection difficulties.
- ○ Prostate problems. Your main risk is benign (i.e. non-cancerous) enlargement of the prostate, a condition known as 'BPH' (see page 240).
- ○ Weight. Metabolic changes make it easier for you to pile on the pounds.

YOUR HEALTH PRIORITIES

- ○ Quit smoking.
- ○ Drink alcohol. Seriously! For men over 40, a drink or two a day (but no more) can reduce the risk of heart disease.
- ○ Exercise regularly.
- ○ Eat plenty of fresh fruit and vegetables and less fat.
- ○ Keep your weight at a safe, healthy level.
- ○ Talk to friends, or perhaps a counselor, about feelings of anxiety or depression.
- ○ Be vigilant for the signs of potential health problems.

YOUR REGULAR HEALTH CHECKS

(for all 45–59-year-olds)
- ○ Blood pressure (high blood pressure is a risk factor for heart disease): every two years.
- ○ body-mass (your weight/height ratio): every month (see page 58).
- ○ Bowel cancer (by checking a stool sample for blood): every year.
- ○ Cholesterol (a high level is a risk factor for heart disease): every two years.
- ○ Dental examination: every year.
- ○ Eye examination: every year (whether or not you wear glasses or contact lenses).
- ○ HIV: only if you feel you have been at risk and want to know for sure.
- ○ Prostate enlargement (by digital rectal examination and a blood test): if there are symptoms. If not, discuss the merits of an annual screen with your doctor.
- ○ Sexually transmitted infections (except HIV): if there are symptoms. If not, and you are sexually active and changing partners, consider an annual check.
- ○ Skin cancer: examine yourself (or ask a friend) every two months for changes in mole size, shape, or color and other odd-looking skin growths.
- ○ Testicular cancer: examine yourself once a month (see page 256).
- ○ Urine analysis (for diabetes or a kidney infection): every year.

Mr. Senior Citizen—70 years old

YOUR HEALTH ASSETS

○ Mental decline isn't a normal part of ageing for most people. Your problem-solving skills are still particularly strong and your verbal ability and short-term memory will probably remain unchanged well into your 80s.

○ If you haven't developed heart disease by now, your risk of developing it in the future will soon start to fall.

○ Your muscles still have great potential: if you start training, an increase in strength of over 20 per cent is perfectly possible; you'll also lower your blood pressure and create a more positive mental outlook.

YOUR HEALTH RISKS

○ Cancer. This is primarily a disease of old age. Watch out for the main symptoms (see page 226).

○ Dementia. About 10 per cent of people aged over 65, and 20 per cent of over 75s, are affected to some degree by dementia.

○ Heart disease. Your risk is now at its height.

○ Prostate problems. Over 85 per cent of prostate cancer cases are detected in men over 65, and 40 per cent of men in their 70s are affected by a benign prostate enlargement (BPH). The symptoms for both conditions are similar (see page 240).

○ Sexual problems. Your most significant sexual problem is likely to be erectile dysfunction (impotence). Twenty per cent of men in their 70s suffer from this problem, rising to 30–40 per cent of men in their 80s.

○ Stroke. The third biggest cause of death after heart disease and cancer, the vast majority of cases affect men over retirement age.

YOUR HEALTH PRIORITIES

○ It's vital that you remain as physically and mentally active as possible.

○ Regular aerobic exercise, such as walking, can help maintain your fitness and reduce the risk of heart disease and stroke.

○ Brain-stretching activities can help preserve your mental agility.

○ A healthy diet, including a vitamin and mineral supplement, could boost your immune system, increasing your resistance to a range of diseases.

○ Be vigilant for the early signs of any health problems.
○ It'll also help if you can remain sociable, positive, and optimistic.

YOUR REGULAR HEALTH CHECKS

(for all 60-plus-year-olds)
○ Blood pressure (high blood pressure is a risk factor for heart disease): every year.
○ body-mass (your weight/height ratio): every month (see page 58).
○ Bowel cancer (by checking a stool sample for blood): every year.
○ Cholesterol (a high level is a risk factor for heart disease): every two years.
○ Dental examination: every year.
○ Eye examination: every year (whether or not you wear glasses or contact lenses).
○ HIV: only if you feel you have been at risk and want to know for sure.
○ Prostate enlargement (by digital rectal examination and a blood test): if there are symptoms. If not, discuss the merits of an annual screen with your doctor.
○ Sexually transmitted infections (except HIV): if there are symptoms. If not, and you are sexually active and changing partners, consider an annual check.
○ Skin cancer: examine yourself (or ask a friend) every two months for changes in mole size, shape, or color and other odd-looking skin growths.
○ Testicular cancer: examine yourself once a month (see page 256).
○ Urine analysis (for diabetes or a kidney infection): every year.

The signs of ageing

Scientists still aren't completely sure why our bodies show signs of ageing. One theory, based on evolutionary principles, is that we decline and die once we've reproduced and made our contribution to the gene pool. If we lived forever, we could only continue to supply the same genes, restricting the capacity of our species to adapt successfully to the environment. We'd also be competing for food with our descendants, affecting their ability to reproduce and make their own important genetic contribution. Whatever the explanation for ageing, there's no mistaking the signs.

○ If your genes have so determined, you'll lose much of the hair on your head, a process that can start when you're still in your 20s. A decrease in the number of cells that maintain hair color also means that whatever hair you've got is likely to lighten. Annoyingly, as you age, hair starts sprouting out of your ears, nose, and eyebrows.

TESTING, TESTING

Some health checks you can do easily at home, such as examining your testicles for lumps or your skin for abnormal moles; other tests, like a dental check or a prostate examination, can only be performed by a health professional. But with a growing range of home health-testing kits becoming available, there are many checks for which you have now a choice. Are these do-it-yourself tests really any use?

○ **Cholesterol test**

How does it work? You prick your finger with a sterile lancet and squeeze a few drops of blood into a test meter. The result is read off a thermometer-type scale.

Is it accurate? Yes, if the instructions are followed precisely. But it's also easy to get a false reading; this could be a particular problem if you get an inaccurate low result.

○ **Blood-pressure monitor**

How does it work? You attach a cuff to your wrist, press a button to inflate it and then read off your blood pressure on the display.

Is it accurate? Tests show not all monitors are accurate. They're probably of use only to people already known to be suffering from high blood pressure.

○ **Urine test**

How does it work? You hold a thin strip of card in your urine stream and compare the colored sections to a chart. Abnormalities could be a sign of diabetes.

Is it accurate? A home test might suggest a problem but can't provide a conclusive diagnosis, and there's always the danger of a falsely reassuring result.

○ **Stool test**

How does it work? Dip a collection stick in a stool sample, place in a bottle, and watch the test window for the result. Traces of blood could be a sign of bowel cancer or other diseases of the colon.

Is it accurate? Yes, but the test can't identify the cause of any bleeding—it could be anything from hemorrhoids to cancer. A falsely negative result could be dangerous; a false positive could cause needless anxiety. If you can see blood in your stools, don't waste time testing them—see a doctor soon.

WILL WE EVER LIVE FOR EVER?

Almost certainly not, but the next 20 years should see some key medical developments which will not only make your life healthier and longer but will also change the way you use health services. You can expect to see:

○ Computerized doctors. Your first visit to a clinic could well involve talking to a computer for a preliminary diagnosis. You'll also be able to discuss your problems with a nurse or doctor from home by e-mail and to download reliable information from a vast range of specialist Internet websites.

○ 'Telepresence'. If you need expert advice, your doctor will examine you under the guidance of a specialist linked by a 'videonet'. Online surgeons using 'remote hands' will be able to operate surgical instruments from anywhere in the world.

○ Bio-sensors. Electronic interfaces mounted on your body will monitor your vital signs. If you're about to have a heart attack, you'll be advised (via your wristwatch) to get medical help.

○ Automatic health screens. Smart toilets will check your deposits and warn you of any problems.

○ A male contraceptive pill, enabling men to take greater responsibility for contraception.

○ A cure for the common cold. This could well take the form of a drug contained in a nasal spray that inactivates an enzyme within cold viruses.

○ Injections that don't puncture the skin. Drug particles are propelled at supersonic speed to penetrate the skin without pain or risk of infection from contaminated needles.

○ Edible vaccines—genetically modified fruit and vegetables that immunize against disease. These could be a cheap and easy way to protect people from such illnesses as cholera and hepatitis.

○ A vaccine for HIV/AIDS as well as better treatments for those with the disease.

○ Greater integration of complementary medicine into the mainstream as more scientific studies prove its usefulness.

○ Greater attention paid to the health of men. Health services will become more male-friendly (they will be open for longer, for example, and will increasingly be located where men are—bars, clubs, sporting venues, the workplace, etc.), and there will be more effective healthy-living campaigns aimed specifically at men (e.g. encouraging them to stop smoking, lose weight, etc.).

○ By the time you're 70, you'll have shed over 40 pounds of dead skin cells. Because the turnover rate of skin cells diminishes with age, and the skin naturally weakens, you're increasingly prone to wrinkles.

○ Fat and fluid accumulate under the eyes, causing them to sag; changes in the amount of a skin protein called elastin, combined with shifting levels of fat, create a double chin. Ears will also get larger with age: it's been calculated that, on average, they increase in length by 0.22 mm a year between the ages of 30 and 93.

○ As your blood vessels lose elasticity, your blood pressure could well rise with age. A healthy young adult has a blood pressure of about 110/75—i.e. 110 'systolic' (when the blood is being pushed by a heart beat) and 75 'diastolic' (when the blood is flowing steadily between beats). By the age of 60, this may well have risen to about 130/90. Blood pressure isn't normally considered high until it reaches 160/95.

○ Unless you exercise regularly, your muscle mass will decrease, causing a loss of strength and sagging skin, especially around the arms and shoulders. Between the ages of 30 and 80, your arm-muscle strength could fall by 30 per cent and your leg strength by 40 per cent.

○ Your lungs become stiffer with age, so you can't breathe in as much air. If your lifestyle is sedentary, your maximum breathing capacity may decline by some 40 per cent between the ages of 20 and 70.

○ As men age, they burn off a higher proportion of calories from carbohydrate and a lower proportion from fat when they exercise. This means that older men may have to work out harder and longer to stay trim.

○ Your testosterone levels decline by about one per cent a year after your mid-20s.

○ You'll lose about three per cent of your skeletal weight per decade and, throughout your adult life, the total mineral density of your bones will fall by 15 per cent.

○ After puberty, your immune system slowly becomes less effective and you're increasingly prone to a range of illnesses.

○ You may need glasses or contact lenses as your eye lenses start to harden (typically during your 40s); your ability to perceive colors also falls with age.

○ Your hearing may also be less efficient from the age of about 30; problems usually start with high-pitched sounds.

Many of these changes are inevitable and irreversible, and all we can do is to try to find ways of coming to terms with them. But other changes, to such things as muscle mass, lung capacity, and weight gain, can be held at bay if we lead an active lifestyle and follow a healthy diet.

CHAPTER 4

WORKING IT OUT:
HOW TO BE FIT FOR LIFE

There's one aspect of healthy living many men need no encouragement to take seriously—exercise. Drinking orange juice instead of beer or eating beans instead of beef might seem wimpish to many, but there are no such problems with playing football, going for a five-mile run or humping weights around a gym. For many of us this could be because the fitter we are, the more manly we feel. It's certainly difficult to think of a male super-hero who takes an hour to run a mile or can't lift a dumper truck off the ground with just one hand. But men don't exercise just to feel more masculine: our increasing interest in working out reflects the mounting pressures we feel to look good at a time when it can sometimes seem as if images of lean and muscular men are everywhere. And, of course, a large number of men exercise simply because it feels good.

But some of us are still not active enough to make a difference to our health. Surveys of men in Australia, Canada, the UK, and the USA show that only one-third of adult men are moderately active on a regular basis and just one in 10 is vigorously active. After school or college, our participation in sport can easily decline rapidly—almost before we know it, all we're doing is watching on television what we once loved to play. If we own a car, we probably prefer to drive into town than walk. If we work full-time, live with a partner, or have parental responsibilities, it can seem hard to find the opportunities for regular exercise. By the time we've reached middle age, it's easy to assume that exercise is really only for younger guys and that, if we tried it, we'd soon find ourselves being prepared for open-heart surgery.

In fact, the opposite is much more likely to be the case. It might sound incredible but, despite its undoubted attractions, the lifestyle of a couch potato creates as big a risk of heart disease as smoking a pack of cigarettes every day. An inactive lifestyle has also been linked to a higher risk of stroke, diabetes, colon cancer, osteoporosis, anxiety, depression, memory loss, and low self-esteem. Too many men are missing out on a cheap and reliable health benefit which, if it were a drug, would almost certainly be in far greater demand than Viagra. Fortunately, however, it's never to late to learn to love exercise—and you don't have to become a fitness freak or even buy a jock-strap.

Why bother to exercise?

○ You'll feel better. Exercise often has an almost instantaneous impact, reducing feelings of anxiety, depression, and anger; it can even generate feelings of euphoria. These effects could be due to increased blood flow through the brain, a rise in the concentrations of the brain chemicals noradrenaline and serotonin, and an elevation in the blood level of beta-endorphins, a naturally produced pain killer. Exercise can also provide a welcome, and often lasting, distraction from depressing thoughts.

○ You'll have more energy. Even if you're exhausted after a workout, the chances are you'll experience a 'rebound' effect within a couple of hours—in other words, you'll end up feeling more energized than before you started exercising. This is partly physiological—it's those naturally produced endorphins again—but it could also be because exercise has the psychological effect of making you feel more in control of your life and as if those wearisome tasks you've been putting off are actually manageable after all.

○ You'll cope better with stress. It's believed that because exercise has many of the same physiological properties as stress—they both cause the heart to beat faster, temporarily raise blood pressure and produce sweat—exposure to exercise 'toughens up' the body, making it easier to deal with all stressful situations.

○ You'll look good. Exercise alone isn't enough to give you a body like a Greek god— you'll also need to change your diet—but it can help. The even better news is that even substantial periods of exercise don't have the effect of automatically increasing your appetite to compensate for the extra energy burnt off. So you're not going to feel compelled to run (or crawl) from the gym to the nearest burger joint.

○ You'll have a better sex life. Research suggests that men who work out moderately and regularly experience increased sex drive, more satisfying sex, and fewer problems with erectile dysfunction (impotence). One study even found they had more frequent sexual intercourse and masturbated more, too. This could be related to an exercise-induced boost in testosterone levels and the simple fact that getting in shape boosts a man's self-image and confidence. But do remember to take a shower first if you're hoping for some action between the sheets.

THE SCIENCE BIT

○ Exercise can extend your life. The more energy a man expends each week in vigorous physical activity (such as brisk walking, jogging, or running), the less likely he is to die prematurely from any cause, according to a long-term study of over 17,300 men in the USA. The risk of death is one quarter lower among men who burn off 1500 or more calories a week in vigorous activity compared to those using fewer than 150 calories.

○ It's never too late to start. A study of almost 10,000 men aged 20–82 found that men who were judged unfit at two medical examinations about five years apart had the highest death rate and men who were physically fit at both examinations had the lowest. (In fact, the unfit men were three times more likely to die than the fit men.) But what's particularly significant is that men who changed from being unfit to fit between the two examinations reduced their risk of dying by 44 per cent compared to those men who remained unfit.

○ Exercise is particularly good for the heart. A study of over 7700 middle-aged British men shows that inactive men are not only more likely than active men to suffer a heart attack, they're also about twice as likely to die from it. Regular physical activity helps the heart by decreasing blood clotting and lowering blood pressure; even moderate activity can also produce a 10 per cent fall in the level of 'bad' LDL cholesterol and a six per cent rise in 'good' HDL cholesterol.

○ It cuts your cancer risk. There's very strong evidence that physically active men are much less likely to develop colon cancer than sedentary men. One large US study found that active men run about half the risk.

○ Exercise is good for bones. Couch potatoes are at a higher risk of suffering from osteoporosis in old age. (This is a condition in which the bones thin, become weaker, and are much more likely to break.) One study of over 5000 retired men in California found that those who exercised for less than 30 minutes a day ran twice the risk of a hip fracture than those exercising for one hour or more. Impact-type exercises (e.g. squash, tennis, aerobics, or weight-training) are thought to be particularly effective in increasing bone density and strength.

○ Physical activity helps prevent diabetes. A 14-year study of almost 6000 University of Pennsylvania graduates found that the incidence of diabetes declined by six per cent for each additional 500 calories burnt off each week during physical activity.

THE SCIENCE BIT

○ Exercise reduces stress. In one study, unfit male students were asked to spend 10 weeks taking part in an aerobic fitness program, a relaxation program, or a discussion group. They were then asked to take part in a very stressful (non-physical) competition. The men in the exercise group not only performed better in the test but also experienced significantly less anxiety, depression, and fatigue following the competition than the men in the other two groups. Other research also suggests that unfit people who've experienced lots of stress in the preceding year are considerably more prone to physical illness than fit people.

○ You'll perform more effectively at work. Regular exercisers are generally more alert, have improved powers of concentration, and are better at making complex decisions than non-exercisers. Their morale is often higher and they are less likely to take sick leave.
○ You'll probably live a lot longer—and be healthier and more active for a greater proportion of your life—than someone who has a sedentary lifestyle.

What is fitness?

Although it's pretty obvious that an Olympic athlete is physically a lot fitter than a 280-lb/14-stone), chain-smoking hot-dog salesman, it's not possible to say that any one person is fit while another is unfit. There is no identifiable, single point at which you can pass from a state of unfitness to fitness. Fitness is, in fact, a continuum made up of three 'S' factors: stamina, strength, and suppleness. You become fitter when your performance on one or more of these components starts to improve.

○ Stamina, also known as endurance, aerobic, or cardiovascular fitness, is the single most important element of your fitness. It reflects your ability to keep going without quickly becoming tired or puffed out, and is directly related to the efficiency of your heart—the more stamina you have, the less hard your heart has to work to supply your muscles with oxygen during physical activity.
○ Strength reflects the amount of external force your muscles can exert. It's essential for pulling, pushing, and lifting, not just in the gym but also for carrying the shopping, digging the garden, mixing cement, and attempting some of the rather more exotic sexual positions.

○ Suppleness, or flexibility, concerns the range of motion available at your joints. It's essential for any sport—not least because it protects against injury—and will come in handy when you're crawling beneath your kitchen sink to unblock the waste pipes.

Sports scientists have devised batteries of tests to measure performance on each aspect of fitness. Some experts believe that people beginning a fitness program should have their current level of fitness assessed. It can then be measured again in three or six months to see how much improvement has taken place. But the problem with fitness tests is that they measure performance only on the specific tasks being assessed rather than all-round fitness, they're liable to a wide margin of error, and they can prove demotivating if they suggest incorrectly that only slight improvements have occurred. You're probably better off simply following a straightforward, increasingly demanding exercise program. As you're able to perform a variety of tasks which were previously difficult or impossible, you'll know you're getting fitter.

I'm Mr. Lazy—how can I change?

○ You're more likely to be able to increase your level of physical activity if you're clear and positive about your motives. Do you want to feel and look in good physical shape? Do you want to maintain or improve your health, perhaps because you've been affected by particular problems, such as back pain? Would taking more exercise provide you with a sense of achievement? Could exercise simply be good fun or a way to relax? You're much more likely to give up exercise if you're doing it because you feel you 'should' be working out or you feel guilty if you don't.

○ Setting so-called 'SMART' goals can help with motivation: these are Specific, Measurable, Agreed, Realistic, and Timed.

➲ Specific goals could include being able to walk to the station without getting puffed out, losing some weight, or even joining an exercise class.

➲ Measurable goals might be trimming an inch off your waistline or cycling to work in under 20 minutes.

➲ Agreed goals are those you're committed to for yourself rather than ones other people are trying to impose on you. For example, if you're starting to exercise because your partner wants you to lose weight, even though you're happy as you are, then you probably won't keep going for long.

(43)

➲ Realistic goals are just that. There's no point in deciding to run a marathon next month if you've been a couch potato for the last 10 years; you could more plausibly decide to jog or a mile or two within a month. Whatever your current level of fitness, remember that progress is normally steady but slow: if you're new to exercise, for example, you'll notice quite soon that it's easier to walk up stairs, but it'll probably take a lot longer before you can expect to see the first signs of a six-pack on your abdomen.

➲Timed goals have a deadline rather than being open-ended. You could decide, for example, to get in shape for a 15-mile charity walk in two months' time, or to work toward completing a marathon in 12 months' time.

○ Your initial goal should be to exercise moderately for at least 30 minutes a day for three days a week. Over a few weeks, try to increase this to five days a week—believe it or not, exercising at this level is enough to provide major health benefits, according to the US Center for Disease Control, the American College of Sports Medicine, and the UK Health Education Authority. The even better news is that each 30 minutes of exercise needn't be in one session—it can be accumulated throughout the day in chunks of at least 10 minutes. Moderate exercise includes walking fast or briskly, swimming, table tennis, golf, dancing, heavy DIY (e.g. mixing cement), digging the garden, and heavy housework—in fact, virtually anything that raises the heartbeat and leaves you feeling slightly warm and slightly out-of-breath. You should aim to be exercising at level 3 on the so-called 'scale of perceived exertion' (see page 46).

○ As you get fitter, aim to increase your level of exercise to two or three continuous and vigorous 20–30 minute aerobic workouts each week. (At levels 6–8 on the scale of perceived exertion.) This level of exercise—which includes squash, running, football, fast cycling, tennis, aerobics—provides the optimum health benefits. It should, ideally, be accompanied by additional strength and stretching exercises.

○ Whatever exercise you decide on, you're much more likely to stick with it if you enjoy it. In fact, if your regime includes activities you find pleasurable you're almost certainly much better off exercising moderately over a long period of time than indulging in short-lived bursts of more intense activity that you find tedious.

○ Make time for your exercise. You may need to get up 10 minutes earlier, or take a slightly longer lunch break, to allow time for a walk. If you want to work out on two evenings a week, make a note in your diary so you don't end up booking something else instead.

○ Keep a record of how you're progressing. You could measure improvements in speed, for example, or the distance you're able to cover, the fall in your waist measurement, or the increase in the weights you can lift. Regularly reviewing your progress can provide motivation and enable you to decide your next set of fitness goals.

○ Don't get discouraged if you take a break from exercise. Some research suggests that, if you take just 10 days off, it can take up to 30 days to restore the level of fitness you enjoyed before the break, but the good news is that if you've been fit before it'll be easier for you to regain your fitness than it was for you to achieve it in the first place. One practical tip: if you're about to go on holiday, schedule a work-out in your diary for a day or two after you return. If you don't, it'll probably take you longer to get back into exercise.

○ Don't go over-the-top with expensive equipment. For general exercise, all you need is a decent pair of running shoes, track-suit pants, a tee-shirt, and a pair of tightish underpants to support your personal equipment. A set of dumbbells and a barbell are also useful for strength exercises (but you can also use cans of food, small tins of paint, or plastic bottles filled with water or sand).

Your best route to fitness

Here's a four-stage fitness program covering stamina, strength, and suppleness. Follow this and you'll be well on the way to excellent fitness. Before you start, however, make sure you haven't any medical problems that might make these (or any other) exercises unsafe for you (see page 53).

STAGE 1

A gentle preparatory stage. However fit you are (or would like to think you are), don't skip this. Aim to complete the following three times a week or every other day:

○ Walk briskly for 20 minutes. You should be at level 3 on the scale of perceived exertion.
○ Stretch your calves, quadriceps, and hamstrings after each walk. (See page 51 for details.)

Don't move on to Stage 2 unless you can complete this one comfortably. Repeat Stage 1 as many times as you need to.

THE SCALE OF PERCEIVED EXERTION

To be sure of getting good health benefits from your aerobic exercise, you need to be working at the right level. Some fitness experts recommend exercise at different levels of heart rate; others prefer an easier-to-use method based on a simple scale of how hard the exercise feels. A scale of 0–10 is widely used.

HOW HARD DOES IT FEEL?	LEVEL
Not at all	0
Very, very light	0.5
Very light	1
Light	2
Moderate	3
Somewhat heavy	4
Heavy	5
	6
Very heavy	7
	8
	9
Very, very heavy	10

If you're new to exercise, you should start with moderate-intensity exercise at level 3. As you become fitter, steadily increase your effort until you're working out vigorously at levels 6–8. You should never go above level 8. A good guide is that you should never be exercising so hard or be so out-of-breath that you can't give a reasonable reply to a question.

As you become fitter, you'll have to work harder to maintain your level of perceived exertion. For example, whereas you once had to run at eight miles per hour (mph) to be at level 7, you now find you have to run at 10 mph.

STAGE 2

Aim to complete the following three times a week or every other day:

○ Do a mix of brisk walking and jogging for 30 minutes. (If you're unable to jog, perhaps because of a back or joint problem, substitute cycling or use a stepping, rowing, or cross-country skiing machine.) Don't exceed level 5/6 on the scale of perceived exertion; if you go higher up the scale, slow down straightaway.

○ For the first session, walk for two minutes then jog for one, walk for two, jog for one, etc. (If you're cycling, etc., mix different levels of effort in the same way.)

○ For the second, alternate one minute of walking with one minute of jogging.

○ For the third (and any subsequent) session, alternate one minute of walking with two minutes of jogging.

○ Strength exercises (see page 48 for details):
 ➲ Squats (1 set of 12 repetitions)
 ➲ Push-ups (1 x 12)
 ➲ One-arm rows (1 x 12 each side)
 ➲ Shoulder presses(1 x 12)
 ➲ Abdominal crunches (2 x 12)

○ Stretch your calves, quadriceps, hamstrings, chest, and back.

Don't move on to Stage 3 unless you can complete this stage comfortably. Repeat Stage 2 as many times as you need to.

STAGE 3

Aim to complete the following three times a week or every other day:

○ Do a mix of brisk walking and jogging (or your substitute aerobic exercise) for 40 minutes. Try to spend longer intervals jogging, hopefully working up to alternating one minute of walking with three minutes of jogging. You should still be careful not to exceed level 5/6 on the scale of perceived exertion; if you do exceed it, slow down straightaway.

○ Strength exercises:
 ➲ Squats (1 set of 15 repetitions)
 ➲ Push-ups (1 x 15)
 ➲ One-arm rows (1 x 15 each side)
 ➲ Shoulder presses (1 x 15)
 ➲ Abdominal crunches (2 x 15)
 ➲ Crunch twists (1 x 15 each side)
 ➲ Back extensions (1 x 15)

○ Stretch your calves, quadriceps, hamstrings, chest, and back.

Don't move on to Stage 4 unless you can complete this stage comfortably. Repeat Stage 3 as many times as you need to.

STAGE 4

Aim to complete the following three times a week or every other day:

○ Start with 10 minutes brisk walking, jog for 20 minutes, and then walk for 10. (Or adapt your substitute aerobic exercise in the same way.) Don't exceed level 7/8 on the perceived scale of exertion; if you go higher up the scale, slow down straightaway.

○ The strength exercises should be performed twice, this time as a circuit. In other words, perform all the exercises once and then do them all again in the same order. Start with a 30-second rest between each exercise, but as you progress try and cut down on the rest time until you can do the whole circuit without a break.

   ⮑ Squats (1 x 12)
   ⮑ Push-ups (1 x 12)
   ⮑ One-arm rows (1 x 12 each side)
   ⮑ Shoulder presses (1 x 12)
   ⮑ Dumbbell curls (1 x 12)
   ⮑ Triceps dips (1 x 12)
   ⮑ Abdominal crunches (1 x 15–20)
   ⮑ Crunch twists (1 x 15 each side)
   ⮑ Back extensions (1 x 15)

○ Stretch your calves, quadriceps, hamstrings, chest, and back.

In the following weeks, try to lengthen the jog times and to perform the circuit three times without rest breaks.

The exercises

FOR STRENGTH

○ Squats (to beef up your thigh muscles)
   At first you may need to do these without a weight, either with your arms crossed in front of you at shoulder height or (if you need more support) with your backside against a wall or door. If you use a weight, place a

barbell across your shoulders and behind your neck. However you do your squats, keep your feet shoulder-width apart and, with your back straight, lean forward slightly and lower your backside as if sitting down in a chair. When your thighs are parallel to the floor, push up back to the starting position.

○ Push-ups (for the chest and triceps muscles)
The classic muscle-building exercise. Start with your hands on the floor, level with, but just slightly wider than, your shoulders. Your legs should be straight and their weight supported on your toes. Push up with the arms, keeping your back and legs straight. When your arms are almost fully extended, lower your body until your nose and chest almost touch the floor and then push up again.

○ One-arm rows (strengthens the back)
Put your right knee and right hand on a knee-high bench and keep your left foot flat on the floor. Hold a dumbbell off the floor in your left hand (your left arm should be hanging vertically) and keep your back straight. Without moving your body, pull the dumbbell toward your abdomen by bending your elbow until it's pointing toward the ceiling. Your elbow shouldn't move sideways during the exercise, only up and down. Lower and repeat for both sides of the body.

○ Shoulder presses (works the shoulders)
Sit on a bench, or stand up, with your feet and knees shoulder-width apart. (If you're standing, your knees should be slightly bent.) Hold a dumbbell in each hand at shoulder level with your palms facing forward. Keeping your back straight, push up both arms until they are almost straight. Touch the weights together gently. Your arms mustn't swing out during the exercise. Lower and repeat.

○ Dumbbell curls (for the biceps)
Stand holding a dumbbell in each hand—your hands should be by your thighs and your palms should be facing ahead of you. Keep your arms and back straight, your knees slightly bent and your feet shoulder-width apart. Slowly raise the weights to your chest before returning to the start position.

○ Triceps dips (builds the triceps, unsurprisingly)
To get into the start position, stand in front of, and facing away from, a solid chair. Bend your knees, squat down and place your hands on the edge of the seat of the chair behind you. Your hands should be shoulder-width apart. Your weight should now be supported by your arms, which should be straight. Your knees should be bent at about 90 degrees and

your feet flat on the floor. Now lower your body until your elbows are at 90 degrees and then push up. Your feet must remain stationary throughout and your backside shouldn't touch the floor.

○ Abdominal crunches (to strengthen your abdominal muscles)
Lie flat on your back on the floor with your knees bent at 90 degrees. Cross your arms on your chest, tighten your stomach muscles, keep your lower back pressed into the floor and lift up your head and shoulder blades. (Your head doesn't need to be raised higher than 12 inches off the floor—you stop exercising the abs if it is.) Lower and repeat.

○ Crunch twists (to strengthen your abs even more)
Lie flat on your back with your right knee bent at 90 degrees and your left foot resting on your right knee. Put your left arm flat on the floor and hold your right ear lightly with your right hand. Twist your torso so your right elbow moves toward your left knee. Return to the start position and repeat for the other side.

○ Back extensions (for the lower back)
Lie flat on your stomach with your arms straight and beside your body. Lift up your head and shoulders about 6–9 inches off the ground before returning to the start position.

There are some basic rules you should always follow when performing strength exercises:

○ Always warm up aerobically first.
○ Don't rush the exercise so that you're using momentum rather than strength. Slow down, especially during the lowering phase—this should take about twice as long as the lifting phase. When the weight is fully lifted, don't lock your arms.
○ Take a deep breath before each exercise and exhale during the hard part. Never hold your breath—this will increase your blood pressure.
○ Concentrate on maintaining the correct technique—it's safer and you'll derive greater benefits from the exercise. Remember that any injury will stop you training altogether.
○ Extend the muscle through its complete range of movement.
○ Don't get obsessed with using heavy weights—the weights you use should be sufficient for your muscles to find the exercise hard work during the final two or three repetitions in each set. If you're over-ambitious, it's difficult to do the exercise properly and you're more likely

to injure yourself. If you can't manage the right number of repetitions with the weight, reduce the weight until you can.

○ Don't exercise the same muscles every day—a 48-hour break between strength workouts will give them time to recover and will, in fact, enable them to grow faster.

FOR SUPPLENESS

○ Calf stretch
Stand directly in front of a wall and, keeping your legs straight, place the toes of your left foot on the wall, leaving your heel on the floor. Then lean forward until you feel the stretch. Repeat for the other side.

○ Quadriceps stretch (for the front of the thigh)
Holding onto a chair or wall for support, bend your right knee, grab your foot with your left hand and pull it in to your backside. Keep your left leg slightly bent. Repeat for the other side.

○ Hamstring stretch (for the back of the thigh)
Sit on the floor with your right leg straight out in front of you. Bend your left leg so that your left foot is against the inside of your right knee. Then lean forward over your right leg. Repeat for the other side.

○ Chest stretch
Stand with your right shoulder an arm's length from a pillar or protruding corner of a wall. Grab the pillar or wall with your right hand (about 3–4 inches above shoulder height) and, with your arm held straight, rotate your body away from the support until you feel a stretch on the right side of your upper chest. Repeat for the other side.

○ Back stretch
Lie flat on your back, lift up your knees to your chest and hold them there with both hands.

Some men think stretching's a bit 'girly' and leave it out of their exercise routine. But they're making a big mistake: increasing your flexibility not only increases your range of movement during all your daily activities but it also reduces the risk of injury during exercise itself. Never stretch until you've warmed up thoroughly: if your muscles are cold, they're also brittle and could tear or pull. It's also important to hold each stretch for about 25–30 seconds and never to bounce while stretching.

What about 'alternative' exercises?

When we think of exercise, we normally think of an activity that's intense, fast and furious. There's not necessarily anything wrong with that sort of activity, although it does place the body under considerable stress and can create an increased risk of injury, particularly sprains and strains. For this reason, it's worth considering complementing your workouts with less stressful but undoubtedly effective Eastern forms of exercise.

○ T'ai chi

Although it's related to kung-fu, t'ai chi is in fact a non-combative movement therapy that's excellent for reducing stress and improving posture, balance, breathing, and the flexibility of joints. It can reduce the risk of injury in conventional sport and exercise; some trainers believe it may also improve performance by releasing energy as well as increasing reflex speed and mechanical efficiency. Since t'ai chi can significantly raise your heart rate and oxygen uptake, it provides the additional benefits of a moderately intense aerobic workout.

Although there are five main styles of t'ai chi, they're all based on a series of postures linked by rhythmical and graceful movements. The 'short form' of t'ai chi comprises a series of movements that can be performed in about 10 minutes; the 'long form'—108 movements in all—takes up 30–40 minutes. It's difficult to learn t'ai chi from a book or video so your best bet is to join a class and be prepared for daily practice. Although t'ai chi should be practiced outdoors—for reasons to do with ancient Chinese concepts of 'life energy'— you're allowed to stay inside, and even pull the curtains, until you've mastered the basics.

○ Yoga

There are many varieties of yoga, but it is essentially a system of physical and mental training first developed in ancient India. All forms are excellent for improving flexibility and breathing as well as reducing stress. One form of yoga, 'power yoga' (or *astanga* yoga), involves constant activity and provides both an aerobic and a muscle-building workout. *Hatha* yoga is the most popular form in the West, however; this aims to create a relaxed body and a calm mind. You don't have to be able to put your foot behind your neck or stand on your head for three hours to join a yoga class. As a beginner, you'll simply learn a series of basic *asanas* (postures) and *pranayama* (breathing exercises), and you'll need to practice for at least 20 minutes a day.

ARE YOU FIT TO GET FIT?

See your doctor for advice before starting any program of vigorous exercise if you:

○ Have a heart problem
○ Have high or low blood pressure
○ Have joint problems
○ Take pain killers or any other drugs regularly
○ Have back problems
○ Are either very over- or underweight
○ Are over 40
○ Are prone to headaches, fainting or dizziness
○ Have a resting heart rate exceeding 100 beats a minute. You can check this simply by placing two fingers on the inside of your wrist, counting the number of beats over a 15-second period, and multiplying by four. (N.B. begin the counting with 0 rather than 1: go '0, 1, 2, 3,' etc.)
○ Have any other medical condition that could interfere with your taking part in an exercise program.

Whatever your medical history, take any exercise program slowly. If you experience chest pain, dizziness, or feel faint at any time while you're exercising, stop immediately and consult a doctor. During exercise, you should feel no more than a burning sensation in your muscles, not a sharp pain. If something hurts, stop doing it.

What's stopping you?

I might drop dead with a heart attack

The risk is trivial, perhaps 1 in 500,000 to 1 in a million. Since inactive people are at much greater risk of developing heart disease or dying suddenly than physically active people, for the vast majority of men the risks of being sedentary are far greater than the risks of starting exercise. A 14-year study of over 5500 middle-aged British men showed that men who changed from an inactive to an active lifestyle substantially reduced their risk of heart disease—it was 34 per cent lower than for those who remained inactive. The very unlucky few who do drop dead during exercise probably would have died soon anyway.

I'm not the sporty type

Exercise isn't necessarily the same as sport—it needn't be competitive and, since it's possible to work out pretty comprehensively in your living room, you don't even have to do it in public.

I don't like feeling hot and sweaty

You don't have to. If you're unfit, 30 minutes a day of brisk walking (at about 4 mph or more) is just about the best exercise you can do to get in better shape. It improves cardiovascular capacity and stamina, strengthens the muscles of the legs, pelvis, and lower trunk, and helps improve posture. A study of British postmen who deliver mail on foot found they suffered lower rates of heart disease and diabetes; a separate study of middle-aged and elderly men found that three-and-a-half hours of walking a week at an average pace is sufficient to reduce significantly the risk of death from any cause. What's more, you don't need any special equipment to take up walking, it's safe (so long as you look both ways before crossing roads), and it's also free.

I'm not overweight so I don't need to bother

Fitness is actually a more important predictor of mortality than body-mass, at least according to a study of over 25,000 men by the Cooper Institute for Aerobics Research in the USA. This research found that death rates were similar for moderately and highly fit men in all categories of body-mass index, or BMI (see page 58 for an explanation of BMI). Death rates for men with low fitness levels were also higher regardless of their BMI category. It seems you're better off being fit and having a fat waist than having a small waist and being unfit.

I can't run—I've got a bad back, bad knees, and flat feet

Running's not the only, or necessarily the best, form of exercise for everyone. Cycling, rowing, or using a stepping machine are just as good and, because they're low-impact, much safer.

I haven't got the time

There are probably very few people who genuinely can't find some time to increase their level of physical activity. Could you walk part of the way to work, for example, or take a brisk 10-minute stroll at lunchtime? Could you walk up stairs rather than take the lift? If what's stopping you isn't so much time as feeling tired, it's worth remembering that exercise can actually increase your energy levels, creating more time in which you can be productive.

It's boring

Exercise can be, especially if you don't vary it. (If you do the same exercise all the time you're also at greater risk of an over-use injury.) You could try alternating different activities—walking, running, cycling, rowing, swimming, stepping, etc. Also, if you're doing some weights work, you can alternate the parts of your body you're working on (e.g. one session could focus on your legs, the next on your chest and arms). Setting yourself targets should help (e.g. aiming to increase your cycling by five minutes or one mile each week) and exercising with a friend, or under the supervision of a trainer, could increase your motivation.

THINGS YOU DIDN'T KNOW ABOUT EXERCISE

○ You can't use exercise to 'spot reduce' fat. In other words, repeatedly exercising a muscle won't remove the layer of fat that's covering it. Pavarotti could perform sit-ups for 24 hours a day and still have a belly that casts a shadow over Rome. His best route to a six-pack would be regular aerobic exercise, all-round strength training, and eating a lot less lasagne.

○ Although individuals vary, sports scientists have calculated that 6–7pm is generally the best time to exercise. It's all to do with your internal body clock—your flexibility, speed, and strength are naturally all better in the late afternoon/early evening, your body can do more with less effort, and you're more likely to derive fitness benefits.

○ Although moderate exercise can boost your immune system, exhausting exercise might well deplete it. If you run 60 or more miles a week, your risk of illness is about double that of those running fewer than 20 miles. It seems that about 35–45 minutes of moderate exercise tends to boost immunity, while three hours of exertion reduces immune system effectiveness for at least 6–9 hours after the workout; athletes are particularly at risk of catching the common cold.

○ Sex doesn't affect your exercise performance. Treadmill tests comparing men who'd had intercourse 12 hours earlier with men who hadn't found no measurable differences. The only way sex might have an impact is if you're at it all night and don't get enough sleep.

CHAPTER 5

FROM FAT TO FLAT:
BECOMING HALF THE MAN YOU ARE

Men are increasingly concerned about their weight. And it's not just because of those inanely grinning guys on the front covers of men's health and fitness magazines (even though their chiseled abdomens don't contain enough spare lard to fry an egg). Many of us have realized that walking around looking as if we're nine months' pregnant doesn't just look bad, it's also not very good for our health. On the other hand, of course, there are still many men who believe that worrying about weight and faffing around with scales, tape measures, or calorie counters is really 'women's stuff'. After all, you probably can't remember a film where the good guys take time out from slaughtering terrorists and saving the world to check they haven't put on a few pounds. This helps explain why more than half of us are overweight—and the proportion is increasing by about one per cent a year. But it doesn't have to be like this; we don't have to resign ourselves to the slow but steady creep of so-called 'middle-age spread.' So much is now known about why we put on weight, it's actually easier than ever to start losing it.

Why bother to lose weight?

○ You'll feel better. As you're able to exert greater control over your body size and shape, your self-esteem and self-confidence will rise.
○ You'll have more energy. That's simply because your body won't be using up so much simply carrying itself around.
○ Your penis could start to look longer. It's true—abdominal fat can conceal up to two inches of your todger.

THE SCIENCE BIT

○ Non-obese men generally have healthier hearts. A man with a body-mass index (BMI) of 22 or 23 is about half as likely to suffer from major coronary heart disease as a man with a BMI of over 30, according to a study of over 7700 middle-aged British men. He is also over eight times less likely to develop diabetes. (For an explanation of BMI, see page 58.) Other research suggests that a 20 per cent rise in body weight creates an 86 per cent greater risk of heart disease.

○ Losing weight can lower blood pressure. A study of over 2000 adults aged 35–54 which compared the effects of several non-drug treatments on blood pressure found that losing weight produced the biggest long-term fall. This matters because high blood pressure is a big risk factor for heart disease.

○ Obese men are more likely to develop cancer. There's strong evidence linking obesity to an increased risk of colon cancer, especially in men who are also physically inactive. The risk could be as many as two to three times greater than for other men.

○ Being overweight increases the risk of arthritis. A study comparing patients awaiting hip replacement because of osteoarthritis with similar people from the general population found that obese people were almost twice as likely to need the operation as the non-obese. Obesity also increases the risk of developing arthritis of the knee.

○ The heavier you are, the more likely you are to take sick leave from work. A Swedish study found that obese people had over one-and-a-half times more sickness absence than the general population over the course of a year.

○ Your sex drive will increase. As you lose weight, your testosterone levels will start to rise, boosting your libido and improving your fertility.

○ You'll snore less. Most serious snorers are overweight, and, because a thicker neck squeezes the throat, it could make all the difference if you can go down a collar size.

○ You'll live longer. Incredibly, being overweight is actually a bigger risk factor than smoking for heart disease. Your risk of heart disease, certain cancers, diabetes, gall-bladder disease, and a range of bone, joint, and skin disorders will fall as you lose weight. Assuming you're not underweight, if you can lose 22 pounds, on average you'll reduce your risk of premature death by up to 25 per cent, your risk of developing diabetes will fall by 50 per cent, and your blood pressure will be significantly reduced. A man of any age who weighs 161lb (11½ stone) and is 5 feet 10 inches tall has a 30 per cent lower risk of dying in any given year than a man of the same height who weighs 231lb (16½ stone).

Are you overweight?

In a culture that is obsessed with slimness, it can be difficult to be sure whether or not you are of normal weight, overweight, or obese. One thing at least is clear: you don't have to be as lean as Tom Cruise or Leonardo di Caprio to be healthy. Thankfully, the medics' guidelines are rather more realistic than that.

There are three easy ways of working out whether your health could be at risk:

1. THE WAIST TEST

Your circumference is a good, rough-and-ready indicator of your overall body-fat level. Simply stand up and find your natural waistline (it's mid-way between your lowest rib and the top of the hip bone). Place a tape around this line and take a measurement after relaxing your abdomen by breathing out gently. If you measure 37–39½ inches, you're technically overweight. If your waist tops 40 inches, then you're clinically obese.

2. THE BODY-MASS INDEX

There are two ways to calculate your body-mass index (BMI):

(a) using pounds and inches. Multiply your weight in pounds by 700 and divide that figure by the square of your height in inches. For example, if you're 68 inches tall and weigh 185 pounds, your BMI = 185 x 700 ÷ (68 x 68 = 4624) = 28;

(b) using kilograms and meters. Divide your weight by the square of your height. This means that if you're 1.78 meters tall and weigh 78 kg, your BMI = 78 ÷ (1.78 x 1.78 = 3.2) = 24.4.

Ideally, your score should be between 20 and 25 (in fact, a BMI of about 22 is probably best for long-term health); below 20 and you're underweight; between 25 and 30, you're overweight; and if you're above 30, you're obese. This is the

WEIGHT RANGE (lb)				
Height	Underweight (BMI up to 20)	Healthy weight (BMI 20–25)	Overweight (BMI 25–30)	Obese (BMI 30+)
63 inches	up to 113	113–141	141–169	169 plus
64 inches	up to 115	115–144	144–173	173 plus
65 inches	up to 121	121–151	151–182	182 plus
66 inches	up to 124	124–155	155–186	186 plus
67 inches	up to 127	127–159	159–191	191 plus
68 inches	up to 132	132–165	165–197	197 plus
69 inches	up to 135	135–168	168–202	202 plus
70 inches	up to 140	140–174	174–209	209 plus
71 inches	up to 143	143–178	178–214	214 plus
72 inches	up to 147	147–184	184–221	221 plus
73 inches	up to 151	151–188	188–226	226 plus
74 inches	up to 155	155–194	194–233	233 plus
75 inches	up to 159	159–199	199–238	238 plus

standard test used to check whether your weight could cause health problems. It's not so suitable for fit men with loads of muscle, however, since they could seem overweight even though they're actually carrying very little fat.

3. THE WAIST:HIP RATIO

Measure your waist and hips. (It doesn't matter whether you do this in centimeters or inches.) Measure the circumference of your waist as described in the waist test above; your hips should be measured at their widest part. Divide your waist measurement by your hip measurement to get a ratio. For example, if your waist is 90 cm and your hips 105 cm, the ratio is 0.86. If your ratio is greater than 0.95, you need to lose some weight. This is a particularly useful test because it assesses your fat distribution and calculates whether you've too much around your abdomen.

How do we get fat?

The big question. The big answer is: in more ways than one.

○ We consume more calories than we burn off. The average man needs about 2500 calories a day; if he consumes more, without also increasing his physical activity levels, the so-called 'positive energy balance' will be stored mainly as fat and he'll pile on the pounds.

○ We're couch potatoes. Too little physical activity is probably the single most significant reason why most people put on weight. The use of cars, escalators, electric lawnmowers, and television remote controls has become endemic. Many more men now spend their working days sitting at desks and staring at computer screens; far fewer do work involving any serious level of physical activity.

○ We love fat. Fast-food outlets are everywhere, and ever-increasing numbers of us prefer to stick ready-prepared meals in the microwave oven rather than spend time cooking. Much of this food is high in fat and therefore calorie-dense. (One gram of fat contains nine calories whereas one gram of carbohydrate or protein contains just four.) Most of us get over 40 per cent of our daily calories from fat; ideally, we should be getting 30 per cent or less.

○ It's genetic—for some. A proportion of those who become very overweight seem to have a particular problem with their fat intake. Scientists have identified a hormone (leptin) whose role appears to be to travel from fat deposits around the body to the brain; when these deposits have reached a normal level, leptin tells the brain to stop eating. Research suggests that obese people have high levels of leptin in their blood because they've been born with faulty receptors in their brains, which prevent the 'STOP EATING DONUTS NOW' message getting through. But even if you have a biological susceptibility to weight gain, it's still your consumption of excess calories that's directly responsible for your spare tyre.

I've got five bellies—how can I change?

If you're obese (with a BMI of 30 or more) you should seek expert advice about losing weight. Otherwise, this program should help.

○ Decide you want to lose weight. You're more likely to succeed if you're clear about your reasons and feel well-motivated. You might decide you want to shed some flab so you'll feel more confident at work or more attractive to a potential or current partner. You could already have a health problem—such as back pain or high blood pressure—and know that getting in better physical shape will help your recovery. It's also possible that you want to perform better at a sport or leisure activity and know that being lighter will make a difference. But you're unlikely to lose much weight if you're doing it just to please someone else, such as a partner who's been nagging you for months. It has to be your choice and your decision.

○ Work out what might be stopping you losing weight. It could just be that you don't know how to go about it or that you simply love the foods that are worst for your waist. You might also feel embarrassed about starting to take it seriously because it seems an 'unmanly' thing to do. Once you can identify the problem, it's easier to sort it out. Information is now easy to get hold of. You may have to eat less of your favorite foods, or accept that you'll feel embarrassed for a while, but it'll help if you make a conscious decision that losing weight is ultimately more important to you. Another way to get round the feeling that slimming isn't for blokes is to combine it with a serious commitment to exercise; telling people you're in training might sound less 'wimpy' than whingeing about how your trousers all feel too tight these days.

○ Forget about diets and calories. Severely restricting your calorie intake might help you lose weight in the short term but the odds are you'll bounce back as soon as you come off the diet. What's more, low-calorie diets aren't sustainable for long—you're hungry all the time and obsessed with food—and you simply can't live your life weighing everything you eat and calculating how many calories it contains.

○ Forget about quick-fix gimmicks—they don't work. There's no evidence that special diet drinks, let alone herbal pills or electronic muscle stimulators, can make any long-term difference to your weight. If you do try them, the odds are that the only thing that will be lighter is your wallet.

○ Set yourself a realistic weight target, perhaps something you've weighed in at before (although not when you were 12 years old). Or aim to reduce your beer gut until you can fit into those jeans you've been keeping for old times' sake.

○ Think long-term. A steady loss of one to two pounds a week, or a one per cent per week reduction in waist size, is realistic and sustainable. You shouldn't feel hungry, either.

○ Don't just think food, think physical activity. To lose weight, you need to use more calories than you eat—and a pincer movement on your flab could get better results. Any increase in physical activity will make a difference. So take the stairs rather than the lift, walk to the station rather than use the car, and get up to change channels on your television rather than use the remote. (Scientists have found that even simply staying on your feet and

WHY DIETS DON'T WORK

○ When you cut your calorie intake drastically, your body reacts as if it's being starved and starts conserving energy by reducing your metabolic rate. This means that your rate of weight loss will slow down even if you maintain your diet.

○ Because you're hungry and the diet's so hard to follow, you could easily become obsessed with food, making it hard to concentrate on much else. Indeed, a UK Institute of Food Research study found that a preoccupation with dieting can affect working-memory capacity in a similar way to states of anxiety or depression.

○ You'll probably feel lethargic, making it harder for you to enjoy physical activity—even though that's an excellent way of aiding weight loss.

○ You risk losing muscle as well as fat. This will lower your metabolic rate still further, making it even harder to continue losing weight.

○ You will lose weight but it's very difficult to keep it off if your body's screaming for food because it thinks it's being starved. Sooner or later, you'll give in to temptation and you could well end up overeating or even bingeing. You could then feel guilty, ashamed, and hopeless, and abandon the diet. You might easily end up weighing more than you did before you started.

○ The only sure way to maintain long-term weight loss is to take it slowly and change your eating habits permanently.

fidgeting a lot can be enough to burn off almost 700 calories a day.) But one of the best ways of guaranteeing sustained weight loss is to take up regular exercise. Aerobic activity like brisk walking, cycling, or running will help, as will strength work, which builds muscle and increases your metabolic rate. Even if you don't end up losing much weight, improving your fitness will still boost your health.

○ Eat more carbohydrates and cut down on fats. This is undoubtedly your single best dietary strategy for losing weight. Pound for pound, high-carbohydrate foods contain around half the calories of high-fat grub. What's more, if you eat more carbohydrate, it satisfies your hunger more than fat and suppresses your appetite for longer. Over time, your desire to eat fat could also fall because you'll simply enjoy it less (although you may have to experience some 'cold turkey' first—and not the kind that's left over from Christmas dinner).

Key tips:
➲ Eat more of these low-fat foods:

Fruit	Vegetables and pulses	Other
Apples	Beans	Bread
Apricots	Broccoli	Cereal
Bananas	Cabbage	Pasta
Grapes	Carrots	Rice
Kiwi fruit	Cucumber	
Mangoes	Egg-plant (Aubergines)	Fish
Melons	Lettuce	Seafood
Oranges	Mushrooms	White meat or lean red meat
Pears	Onions	
Pineapples	Peas	Low-fat fromage frais
Plums	Peppers	Low-fat yoghurt
Strawberries	Potatoes	Skimmed (or semi-skimmed) milk
Tomatoes	Zucchini (courgettes)	
Other fruits	Other vegetables	Grilled, baked, or steamed foods

➲ Eat less of these high-fat foods:

Bacon	Cream	burgers)
Biscuits	Custard	French fries (chips)
Butter	Donuts	Fried foods of any sort
Cake	Eggs	Ice cream
Cheese (except	Fatty cuts of red meat	Mayonnaise
cottage)	(e.g. beef) and meat	Milk
Chocolate	products (e.g. pies or	Roasted nuts

➲ Use food labels to your advantage. You need to check the amount of fat, in grams, per 100 grams of food—basically, the lower that figure the better. As a general rule, try to avoid foods with more than 10 grams of fat per 100 grams. But you should also be flexible—if you stuck rigidly to this guideline, you'd never be able to eat cheese or nuts or enjoy the occasional treat.

Here are some examples:

TYPICAL VALUES PER 100g				
	Energy (Calories)	Protein (g)	Carbohydrate (g)	Fat (g)
Cheese (Cheddar)	412	25.5	0.1	34.4
Cottage Cheese	98	13.8	2.1	3.9
Bread (Brown)	218	8.5	44.3	2.0
Corn Flakes	360	7.9	88.6	0.7
Liver paté	316	131	1.0	28.9
Peanuts (roasted and salted)	602	24.5	7.1	53.0
Chocolate (milk)	529	8.4	59.4	30.3

Note: Some labels will give an energy value in kilojoules (kJ) as well as calories (often described as kilocalories). One calorie is equivalent to 4.2 kilojoules.

➲ Eat smaller portions: a good way of doing this is simply to eat off a smaller plate.
➲ Eat more slowly. This will allow time for your body's appetite control mechanism to cut in when you're full, enabling you to avoid a second helping.
➲ Use low-fat margarines instead of butter on bread. Better still, if you're eating the bread with cheese, soup, hummus, or other spreads, cut out the margarine as well. And you don't really need margarine or butter if you're eating toast with baked beans, tomatoes, or eggs.
➲ Switch to fat-free or low-fat dairy products. Stick semi-skimmed or skimmed milk on your cereal or in your tea and coffee. But be careful: it's easy to lose any advantage if you end up eating more because you think you can get away with it.
➲ When eating meat, trim off any excess fat, and remove the skin before eating poultry.
➲ Cook vegetables in stock rather than sautéing them in oil or butter. Have your potatoes baked or boiled but not fried or roasted. If you're sticking a filling in a baked spud, there's no need to add butter or margarine first.
➲ Don't add butter or margarine to vegetables before you eat them. As long as you haven't boiled them into a mush, their natural taste should be good enough.
➲ Use oil-free salad dressings, such as balsamic vinegar or plain lemon juice.

- Eat fruit for dessert rather than a cake or pudding. Replace ice cream with frozen fat-free yoghurt or sorbet.
- Keep an emergency supply of low-fat snacks handy to tackle hunger pangs. Apples, pears, and medium-ripe bananas are especially good at keeping you feeling fuller.
- Take your own lunch to work so you have more control over what you eat.

- Don't try to cut out all fats. For a start, you'll never be able to do it unless you become completely obsessive about everything you eat. Secondly, your body actually needs some fats to function: they carry important vitamins, for example, and help produce key hormones. And thirdly, a largely fat-free diet would be so lacking in flavor you'd probably end up bingeing on cream cakes within a week.
- Eat less food more often. This will not only stop you getting hungry (and then eating too much), it will also increase your overall metabolic rate, enabling your body to burn off more calories even when you're lying in bed or watching television. This was demonstrated in a Canadian study which compared the effect on metabolism of food consumed in one large meal with four small meals eaten at 40-minute intervals. Not only did the regime of small meals increase the metabolic rate, it also resulted in the body burning off more fat. As a general rule, never go for more than four hours without eating.
- Always eat breakfast. Not only will it stave off mid-morning hunger pangs for fatty snacks but, if you opt for a high-carbohydrate cereal breakfast, you'll help tilt your overall daily intake of carbohydrate and fat into the right balance. What's more, you're much less likely to develop hemorrhoids or anal fissures— a study conducted at Birmingham University in the UK found that non-breakfast-eaters are 7.5 times more likely to develop these particular pains in the backside.
- Watch what you eat when you drink alcohol. Because your self-control goes down, you can easily find yourself noshing on peanuts or tucking into a late-night pizza or burger. Don't booze before you eat either. A Dutch study in which men and women were given either an alcoholic drink or a range of different non-alcoholic drinks 30 minutes before lunch found that those consuming alcohol ate more calories, ate at a faster rate, ate for longer, and took more time to feel satisfied.
- Consider keeping a 'food diary'. Research shows that people tend to underestimate the amount of high-fat, unhealthy food they eat. If you keep a record of exactly what you eat, you can then check it more carefully to see how much fat it contains. Moreover, if you simply find it tough to make changes, also

IS ALCOHOL FATTENING?

It's certainly high in calories. Pure alcohol contains seven calories per gram, and 98 per cent of what we drink is absorbed by the body (virtually no alcohol actually escapes in the breath or through urine). That means that when we drink a pint of beer, we're adding 170–200 calories (the exact amount depends on the strength) to our daily intake. A 125 ml glass of red wine adds 90 calories, a 25 ml shot of spirits adds 55 calories and a 25 ml glass of liqueur 60 calories.

But because alcohol is essentially a toxin which the body tries to eliminate as quickly as possible, the calories from alcohol itself aren't usually converted into fat. The body prioritizes their use as fuel and burns them off first, leaving the calories from your food and non-alcoholic drinks to be dealt with later. Once your alcohol calories have been eliminated, your body will then store as fat any excess calories from other sources. In a literal sense, therefore, alcohol isn't fattening but if it contributes to an overall positive energy balance (i.e. more calories than you need each day for your activities), you will put on weight.

If you want to lose weight, your best bet is probably not to stop drinking altogether (changing your diet and stopping drinking at the same time may be asking rather too much), but to cut down to a moderate and safe level (see Chapter 7). You can also try 'trading off' alcohol—in other words, in exchange for a pint of beer, cut out a bar of chocolate or go for a 20-minute cycle ride.

writing down when you eat could help you spot where you're going wrong and to decide on changes (e.g. replacing that afternoon Danish pastry with an apple).

○ Change negative 'self-talk'. Do you have an 'inner Marlon Brando', a fat bloke who sits inside your head saying 'You'll never lose weight' or 'You must have some chocolate fudge cake *now*'? Registering these automatic thoughts could enable you to replace them with logical statements that will make a difference, so try telling yourself 'Yes, changing my diet might be tough but it's certainly not impossible.'

○ Don't panic if you lapse. Because weight loss is about making long-term changes, having the occasional blow-out isn't a problem. Don't be too inflexible either. A regime of strict self-control might well work in the short term but is more likely to be undermined by stressful events. If you're less rigid—perhaps eating some chocolate or ice cream once a week—then you're more likely to be able to lose weight in the long term.

What's stopping you?

I can't help being overweight—I've got a slow metabolism

Sorry, but this is one of the biggest myths around. The idea is that lean people have a mechanism for burning off excess calories as heat—scientists call this theory 'adaptive thermogenesis'. The Dunn Clinical Nutrition Centre in the UK tested this by persuading groups of lean and overweight men to live for seven months in conditions in which their diet could be carefully monitored. Even though they were all overfed with 50 per cent more calories than their bodies needed, regular measurements of weight gain, body composition, and energy expenditure revealed no differences between the thin and fat men. The lean men put on as much weight as the fat ones and there was no evidence of any process in which the extra energy was burnt off.

I'll lose some weight when I'm older, when it could really make a difference to my health

Being overweight is a health risk factor at any age, although it's true that the health risks increase when combined with age. But you should remember that because your muscle mass decreases and your metabolism naturally slows down as you get older, the longer you put off losing flab, the harder it'll be.

I couldn't deal with stress without eating

It may well feel that way, but you could be creating a vicious circle in which your anxiety about eating and being overweight in turn creates more stress. Stuffing yourself with sugary foods could also increase your stress by causing rapid swings in your blood sugar and energy levels. Also, your eating is an attempt to soothe the symptoms of stress, not deal with its causes, a much better long-term strategy. There are also many other much less risky stress-reduction techniques you could try (see Chapter 10).

I'm eating much less fat and I'm exercising more but I'm still not losing weight

Your problem could simply be that you're still eating too many calories, even if more of them are from carbohydrate rather than fat. Whatever you eat, if you consume more calories than you burn off, you'll put on weight. Rather than changing the balance of your diet any further, you could try eating smaller quantities of food at meals, drinking less alcohol, and cutting out any high-calorie snacks. If you can't work out where the excess calories are coming from, consider keeping a food diary to help you analyze exactly what you're eating.

WHAT ABOUT SUGAR?

Fat is Public Enemy Number One in the war against flab. It's calorie-dense and difficult to resist. But it's also worth paying some attention to sugar: although it's a carbohydrate (and so, gram for gram, contains less than half the calories of fat), it contains only 'empty' calories—in other words, it lacks nutritionally important stuff like vitamins and minerals. It also increases the body's level of a hormone called insulin, excessive amounts of which inhibit the use of fat as an energy source. Sugar might taste good, but it doesn't do much for us apart from provide a short-term energy boost. And it's easy to eat a lot of sugar without realizing it—in soft drinks, jams, cookies, and confectionery—which can significantly boost our overall calorie intake.

If you like sweet foods, you're more likely to lose weight if you reduce your intake rather than set yourself the impossible goal of giving them up altogether. Fortunately, your taste buds can adjust quite quickly to a reduction in sugar, so what seemed normal will soon taste unpleasantly sweet.

Key tips:
- Switch to a sugar-free breakfast cereal and add your own sugar (but less and less over time).
- Add progressively less sugar to your tea and coffee.
- Choose unsweetened fruit juices rather than ones with added sugar.
- Use savory spreads on bread rather than jam.
- Buy tinned fruits that are in juice rather than in syrup.
- Add less sugar to your cooking.
- Experiment with artificial sweeteners. Some research shows they can help long-term weight loss although they won't change your underlying taste for sweet foods. If you have an unstoppable desire for cola, always go for the low-calorie or diet versions. The regular varieties contain about 35 grams (seven teaspoons) of sugar in a 330 ml can—that's 140 calories. A can of diet cola contains no more than a couple of calories.

A final tip: if you want to increase the amount of fat your exercise burns off, work out before breakfast. Swiss research has found that about 50 per cent more fat is utilized—it's probably because the overnight fast has resulted in low levels of blood sugar, and the body therefore has to draw on more fat for energy.

My problem is that I need to put on weight rather than lose it

If you've been losing weight for no obvious reason, you should see a doctor for a check-up. If you know you've become underweight because of illness, ask your doctor to refer you to a dietitian for some expert advice. But if you're normally underweight—with a body-mass index below 20—and you want to bulk up, you shouldn't start by eating loads of high-fat foods. You might well put on weight that way but it could be at the expense of furred-up arteries.

Key tips:
- ⟳ Always eat at least three meals a day, including breakfast, and eat bigger portions than normal. Increase your carbohydrate intake by basing your meals on bread, pasta, rice, or cereals.
- ⟳ Go for (healthy) between-meal snacks, e.g. fresh or dried fruit or high-energy sports bars.
- ⟳ Supplement your food with high-carbohydrate, low-fat liquids, e.g. fruit juices.
- ⟳ Start an exercise program to increase your muscle mass.
- ⟳ Aim to gain up to two pounds a month.

THINGS YOU DIDN'T KNOW ABOUT WEIGHT

- ○ Spicy foods could help boost your metabolic rate, helping you to lose weight. (The metabolic rate is a measure of how quickly your body burns calories to produce energy.) When Australian scientists injected rats with capsaicin, an ingredient found in chillies and peppers, they found that their large muscles used more oxygen, more energy was used up, and that there was ultimately a decrease in body fat.
- ○ Eat different foods. If the body regularly consumes foods with which it's familiar, the metabolic rate is lower than if it has to digest something new. But if you just can't stop eating the same old stuff, at least try to drink some coffee. Some studies suggest that three to four cups a day can result in a significant increase in metabolic rate.
- ○ An average sauna session produces a one per cent weight loss (that's almost two pounds for a 12-stone man). Unfortunately, most of this is water—you'll probably lose a liter of sweat every 15 minutes—and only the smallest slither of flab will melt away.

CHAPTER 6

WHAT'S COOKING?
THE BEST FOOD—ON A PLATE

Men are increasingly realizing that good health and a good diet are about as inseparable as Laurel and Hardy, Batman and Robin, or R2-D2 and C-3PO, the robots in *Star Wars*. We're beginning to understand that too many breakfast fry-ups, take-away burgers, cookies, and chocolate bars won't do much either to improve our hemorrhoids or to increase our chances of collecting a pension. But it can still be hard for us to change our eating habits. For starters, the unhealthiest foods are usually the ones that taste good and provide all-round satisfaction. Most of us have also grown up believing that men aren't supposed to worry about what they eat and drink. It's all basically fuel, the stuff that keeps us going so that we can do what really matters— work, play football, and have lots of sex. Fretting about whether we're eating enough apples or cabbage, or putting too much salt on our fried eggs, is basically 'sissy' stuff.

The good news is that we don't have to stop eating the foods we like. All we need do is get them into the right balance by eating more fruit, vegetables, and carbohydrates like pasta, rice, and potatoes. By better understanding what makes up a good diet, and making a few simple changes to what we stick in our mouths, we can not only improve our health but also start to enjoy a wider variety of nutritious and tasty foods. It's worth remembering, too, that it's difficult to develop a muscular, well-defined body without eating an extremely healthy diet.

Why bother with a healthier diet?

○ You'll have more energy. A diet rich in 'complex' carbohydrates (e.g. cereals, pasta, potatoes, rice) should provide you with consistent blood-sugar levels and energy throughout the day. Too much fat, on the other hand, can make you feel sleepy, while consuming too much pure sugar (a 'simple' carbohydrate) will cause large blood-sugar swings and sharp fluctuations in energy.

○ You'll feel in a better mood. A high-carbohydrate diet boosts the brain's production of serotonin, a key neurotransmitter that can increase your sense of well-being.

○ You'll look better. A good diet will help you lose weight and improve the health of your skin, hair, nails, and teeth.

○ Your bowels will be grateful. Eating more fruit, vegetables, and cereals will help keep your bottom-end movements smooth and regular.

○ You'll sleep better. Cutting back on caffeine should make it easier for you to fall asleep and sleep through the night.

○ Your immune system will be stronger. A diet rich in fruit and vegetables helps maintain vigorous immune functioning, helping to reduce your chances of developing a wide range of everyday and more serious illnesses.

○ You'll live longer. Up to 35 per cent of cancer cases are believed to be diet-related, and eating more fruit and vegetables, as well as less meat, fat, and salt, could significantly lower the risk. The same changes will also reduce your chances of developing heart disease.

What should I be eating?

Ignore the complicated, confusing, and obsessive diets you'll find in many magazines and books, and don't worry if you're not a nutritional scientist or a cordon-bleu chef. Just try to follow these basic and simple rules:

EAT MORE:

○ Fruit and vegetables. Each day, you should aim to eat five or more apple-sized portions of a variety of fruits and vegetables. (Don't include potatoes in this calculation, even though they should also be a regular part of your diet.)

○ Carbohydrate-rich food. Try to eat seven or more portions of high-carbohydrate (also called 'starchy') foods a day, including bread, cereals, pasta, rice, legumes/pulses, and potatoes.

○ Water. Aim to drink two or three litres (four or five pints) a day (in addition to tea, coffee, and alcohol). Your best guide to whether you're drinking enough is the color of your urine: it should be pale, not dark. Once you're thirsty, you're already dehydrated.

EAT LESS:

○ Fatty food. Although some fat is essential, most of us eat far too much, not

THE SCIENCE BIT

○ Men who eat fruit at least twice a day run one-third of the risk of developing lung cancer than those eating fruit less than three times a week, according to a study of over 34,000 Californians. Other studies suggest that people eating 5–20 servings of fruits and 5–20 servings of vegetables each week also have about half the risk of stomach cancer.

○ The more red meat you eat, the more likely you are to develop bowel cancer. One study of almost 48,000 American men found that those eating beef, pork, or lamb as a main dish five or more times a week were three-and-a-half times more likely to suffer from bowel cancer than men eating these foods less than once a month. This disease is also associated with eating too few vegetables.

○ Although the scientific evidence is as yet inconclusive, several studies suggest that high-fat diets (especially those high in animal fats) increase the risk of prostate cancer. One investigation of over 350 men in the US found that those aged 68–74 who ate the most fat were much more likely to develop an aggressive type of prostate cancer.

○ If you eat fresh fruit every day you're running a 24 per cent lower risk of dying from heart disease, and a 32 per cent lower risk of dying from a stroke, than someone who eats fresh fruit less than once a day, according to a study which compared the death rates of over 10,000 British vegetarians and other health conscious people with the national averages.

○ Elderly men who eat beef at least three times a week run twice the risk of dying from heart disease compared to non-beef-eaters, according to a large study of men in California. The same research found that men and women who eat mostly white bread rather than whole-wheat bread are at almost twice the risk of suffering a non-fatal heart attack.

○ Eating too much salt can cause a potentially dangerous rise in blood pressure (increasing the risk of heart disease and strokes), according to a wide range of studies. Systolic blood pressure can rise by up to 10 mmHg for every extra teaspoon of salt consumed on a daily basis. This matters: while a systolic blood pressure of up to 130 mmHg can be considered normal, over 140 is borderline high and 160 is definitely high. A high-salt diet also increases the risk of stomach cancer.

least because fast foods and convenience foods are stuffed with it. See the 'Fat Facts' box that follows for more detail on the different types of fat, and page 63 for tips on cutting down on how much fat you eat.

○ Protein. Forget the idea that 'grown men' have to eat sides of beef to stay healthy. Sure, protein's a vital nutrient (used for the growth and repair of tissues), but most of us over-estimate how much we need, eat too much, and put on weight because the excess is stored as fat. The average man needs no more than a normal portion of meat or fish plus some bread, rice, pasta, or potatoes.

○ Meat. You don't need to become a vegetarian, let alone a vegan, but you should try limiting your intake of red meat (i.e. beef, lamb, pork, and veal) to no more than two medium slices of pork, three slices of lamb or a five-ounce (raw weight) grilled steak a day.

○ Salt. The World Health Organization recommends a daily intake of six grams (about one heaped teaspoon), well below the current average. Your best bet is to stop adding it to food, whether at the table or during cooking. Since more than half of the salt in our diet comes from manufactured food, eating less tinned or processed food will also help enormously.

○ Sugar. It contains no vitamins or minerals, contributes to weight gain, and can fill us up to the point where we don't feel like eating other, more nutritious food. Watch out for larger-than-you'd-expect amounts in low-fat or fat-free foods (where it's often added to improve flavor) and soft drinks. (For tips on reducing your sugar intake, see page 68.)

○ Caffeine. Too much can make you jumpy and anxious and can interfere with sleep. (See page 79 for more about reducing your caffeine intake.)

○ Alcohol. Aim to consume no more than two drinks a day (see Chapter 7).

What about nutritional supplements?

Wander into any supermarket or pharmacy and you'll find a bewildering choice of pills and potions. Whether or not they can actually improve your health is debatable, but just trying to select a nutritional supplement could be enough to give you a serious headache.

Unless you live on a diet of burgers, burgers, and burgers, you're very unlikely to be at risk of the disorders caused by a vitamin or mineral deficiency. (These include the likes of scurvy, beriberi, and anemia.) Many people now regard taking a daily tablet containing all the major vitamins and minerals as a useful insurance policy, although it's almost certainly unnecessary if you're following all the dietary recommendations in this chapter. The key question is whether there are health benefits from artificially adding nutrients to a diet already good enough to avoid any deficiency problems.

THE FAT FACTS

Fats come in many different forms with strange names that don't give you much of a clue about what's really in them and whether they're okay to eat. Here's what you need to know:

○ **Saturated fat—proceed with caution.** You'll find this in butter, lard, cheese, meat, egg yolks, palm oil, and coconut oil. It's commonly used in cakes, cookies, and pastry. More than any other kind of fat, saturates increase the level of 'bad' cholesterol in the blood and so contribute to furred-up arteries and heart disease.

○ **Trans fatty acids (TFAs)—take care.** Most TFAs are manufactured industrially and added to processed foods such as margarine, cookies, pies, and cakes. (They're also known as hydrogenated or partially hydrogenated vegetable oils.) TFAs act like saturated fats in the blood, and, although they don't do quite as much damage, you should try to limit your intake.

○ **Monounsaturated fatty acids—a good bet.** You'll find this in olive and rapeseed oils, avocados, nuts, and seeds. Most forms of monounsaturated fat have no effect on cholesterol, but if it's in the form of oleic acid (found in olive oil) it can actually lower 'bad' cholesterol levels.

○ **Polyunsaturated fatty acids—the best a man can get.** These show up in most vegetable oils, fish oils, and oily fish. They include two essential fatty acids: Omega-6 (sunflower oil is a very good source) and Omega-3 (found in such fish as sardines, mackerel, and salmon, walnuts, soya-bean and rapeseed oils). Polyunsaturated fatty acids can reduce the risk of heart disease by lowering cholesterol levels.

Remember: all fats are very high in calories, so you'll probably need to cut down your overall intake whatever type of fat you use. If you fry food—and you should try to do so as little as possible—always use a liquid vegetable oil (and not much of it).

ANTIOXIDANTS

Recent research has focused on the so-called antioxidants—mainly the carotenoids (especially beta-carotene, which the body converts naturally to vitamin A), vitamins C and E, and the minerals selenium and zinc. Many studies have shown that these micronutrients can help the body neutralize toxic molecules known as oxygen-free radicals. These are a by-product of our normal metabolism, but our bodies also absorb them from tobacco smoke, exhaust emissions, and other pollutants. We remain healthy so long as the level of free radicals doesn't surge out of control. If it does, free radicals can damage or even kill the body's cells as well as affect blood vessels, and can play a role in the development of cancer and heart disease.

There's mounting evidence that men consuming higher than normal levels of antioxidants are less likely to suffer from these problems:

- One study of 40,000 men aged 40–75 found that those with the highest intakes of vitamin E, achieved through supplementation, were about 40 per cent less likely to develop heart disease than those with the lowest intakes.
- When over 29,500 people in China were given a daily supplement of beta-carotene, vitamin E, and selenium, there was a 13 per cent reduction in all cancer deaths.
- Other research suggests that vitamin E supplements can increase the efficiency of the immune system and that extra intakes of this vitamin, as well as of zinc and selenium, can improve male fertility.

Here's how to increase your intake of the key antioxidants:

ANTIOXIDANT	EAT MORE	SUPPLEMENT (DAILY)
Beta-carotene	Carrots, sweet potatoes, pumpkin, green leafy vegetables, broccoli	9–12 mg
Vitamin C	Fresh citrus fruits, peppers, guavas, sprouts, broccoli, Brussels, cabbage, papaya, kiwi	150–200 mg
Vitamin E	Wheat germ, vegetable oils, soya beans, whole grains, eggs, green leafy vegetables	60–100 mg
Selenium	Brazil nuts, brewer's yeast, wheat germ, tuna, onions, seeds	50–60 micrograms

Lycopene, another antioxidant carotenoid, could be particularly important for men. (Lycopene gives tomatoes their red color and it's also found in pink grapefruit, guava, and watermelon.) A study of over 47,000 men found that those consuming more than 10 servings a week of tomatoes, tomato sauce, tomato juice, and pizza had a 35 per cent lower risk of developing prostate cancer than men eating fewer than one-and-a-half servings a week. Although the link with prostate cancer has not yet been fully proven, it's certainly worth eating more tomato-based foods.

FOLIC ACID

This simple B vitamin—found in leafy green vegetables, liver, orange juice, and whole grains—is now exciting almost as much scientific interest as the antioxidants. The theory (although it's not yet been proved conclusively) is that folic acid lowers the body's level of a substance called homocysteine, an amino acid produced as a natural part of the metabolic process. At high levels, homocysteine can have a toxic effect on the cells and tissues of arteries. It causes scars to which cholesterol can stick, triggering the process that leads to furred-up arteries and heart disease.

○ A Europe-wide study of over 1500 people found that those with the highest homocysteine levels were as likely to develop furred-up arteries as if they smoked 20 cigarettes a day.
○ A UK study found that simply eating a bowl of breakfast cereal fortified with 200 micrograms of folic acid every day for 24 weeks lowers homocysteine levels by 10 per cent.

If you're convinced, you should aim to consume 350–400 micrograms of folic acid a day. Since folic acid is vulnerable to cooking, your best bet is to take a synthetic supplement.

GARLIC

Many scientists claim that garlic not only tastes good but also reduces the risk of a range of diseases. But do the health claims really add up, or should we give them the same wide berth as we would a five-cloves-a-day man?

○ The strongest evidence concerns heart disease. One study of 80 people showed that 16 weeks of treatment with garlic-powder tablets reduced cholesterol levels by 11 per cent and reduced blood pressure by almost 20 per cent.
○ Garlic may also reduce the risk of cancer. A Chinese study of over 1500 people found those eating most garlic and onions (plants that are related) ran only 40 per cent of the risk of stomach cancer compared to those eating the least.

If you want to take enough garlic to make a difference, one to two cloves in food every two days plus a daily supplement of 4–8 mg should be sufficient. Smelly breath is probably an inevitable side-effect, but regular consumption is supposed to lead to a reduction in odor over time.

I don't even know where the kitchen is— HOW can I change?

○ Be sure you want to. You've probably been eating your current diet for years—in other words, it's become a habit. It's difficult to break habits unless you're very committed and have a clear sense of why you're doing it. Rather than changing your diet simply because you've decided to improve your health—a worthy but rather vague objective—it might help to choose some more measurable goals, such as losing some weight, having more energy, or helping to tackle a particular health problem (perhaps you're always getting colds or suffer from constipation).

○ Rather than go for the 'big bang' approach and change your diet completely overnight, think about how you can make a series of small but significant changes. Make a few changes each week until you've put in place the diet you want and feel you can stick to.

Key tips:

➲ Have some fresh fruit with every meal. For breakfast, you could slice a banana, melon, pear, or strawberries on your cereal; you can follow whatever you eat for lunch or dinner with an apple or orange.

➲ If you just can't resist fry-ups for breakfast, have one rasher of bacon, one sausage and one egg rather than two of each; better still, cut out even more fat by grilling the meat, poaching the egg, and having it on dry toast rather than fried bread.

➲ If you always eat a cake for your mid-morning or mid-afternoon snack, try substituting some fresh fruit.

➲ If you normally eat meat every day, try changing to fish every other day. When choosing meat, opt for chicken or turkey (they're lower in fat than red meat). You could also replace some or all of the meat in soups, casseroles, or stews with a tin of beans.

➲ Increase your vegetable consumption by adding a mixed side salad to your lunch or dinner, or including two portions of vegetables in your main meals, either on their own or in soups, stews, pies, curries, or sauces. Stick some salad (cucumber, lettuce, watercress, or tomato) in sandwiches, too.

➲ If you find it hard to cut down on salt, try a low-salt product. Use pepper, herbs, and spices to provide alternative sources of flavor.

➲ If you're addicted to caffeine, don't try cutting back drastically overnight, (unless you want a few days of flu-like withdrawal symptoms). Aim to reduce your daily intake by just one or two cups each week.

➲ Increase your water consumption by remembering to drink a glass or two before every meal. This could also help fill you up, enabling you to eat less.

○ Always eat breakfast. You might prefer to eat your pillow first thing in the morning, but there's no doubt that breakfast is the most important meal of the day. You won't have eaten for up to 12 hours and your blood-sugar levels will have fallen. A meal will help restore them and boost your mood and concentration for the morning. If you have a cereal- or toast-based breakfast, it's highly likely that your meal will be very high in carbohydrate and low in fat, giving you the chance to be a bit more relaxed about the carbohydrate-fat balance during the rest of the day.

○ Plan ahead. If you've got to eat right now and you've next to nothing in your cupboard or refrigerator, you'll probably end up scoffing whatever's there, even if it's a tub of ice cream. You'd be much better off keeping a big enough stock of the food you do want to eat. And here's a top tip: shop for groceries only after eating—if you're hungry, you're much more likely to buy food you don't really want or need.

○ Be tactical. If you're prone to snacking when you're on the move, try and carry with you a supply of fresh or dried fruit. It beats rushing into a shop for a chocolate fix.

○ Experiment. You'll find it much harder to change your diet if you simply try to cut out what's unhealthy rather than finding ways to replace it with something that's tasty as well as better for you. A healthy diet can be much more than a baked potato and a bean salad every day, and there are many fruits besides apples, oranges, and bananas.

Key tips:

➲ Set yourself the target of trying a couple of new foods a week. If you like potatoes, try sweet potato. If you fancy a salad, don't just base it on lettuce— try adding spinach and watercress. If you're partial to tinned tuna, consider tinned salmon for a change. When you next go shopping, spend more time looking at what's on the shelves you normally ignore.

➲ Try preparing a meal you haven't had before once a week. You may have to buy a recipe book for new ideas. If you do, and you're not into cooking, don't waste your time on a cookbook that's aimed at the food-obsessed; go for one that tells you how to throw together basic, healthy grub in under 30 minutes.

➲ Motivate yourself to spend more time in the kitchen by regularly inviting people round for dinner. This could also encourage you to research new dishes.

- ➲ If you can't be bothered to cook, try lower-fat ready meals (they're increasingly available).
- ➲ Eat out in restaurants you don't normally visit to get new ideas about food. If you always eat Italian, try Lebanese or Chinese for a change.

Should I cut back on tea and coffee?

Unless you're a hardened caffeine junkie, you'll know that a strong coffee can give you a buzz. Your heart rate and blood pressure go up, you breathe faster, and you feel more alert. Caffeine 'works' by fitting into brain receptors designed for a naturally occurring tranquilizer chemical called adenosine. By overriding the effects of adenosine, caffeine forces the body to stay in overdrive.

- ○ Just 150–250 mg of caffeine—about two to three cups of percolated coffee—is enough to stimulate the nervous system within an hour and for up to four hours.
- ○ 370 mg a day can be sufficient to cause a wide range of withdrawal symptoms, including tiredness, irritability, and a thumping headache, if caffeine use is abruptly limited or discontinued.
- ○ 500–600 mg a day can easily cause feelings of anxiety and restlessness and interfere with sleep. It's also likely to have a diuretic effect: in other words, it stimulates the kidneys and dehydrates the body.
- ○ At levels of 800 mg a day and upwards, caffeine can may make you feel chronically anxious and irritable; you may even experience muscle tremors and headaches.
- ○ Reassuringly, a fatal overdose of caffeine is almost impossible: you'd have to drink between 50 and 160 cups of instant coffee within 30 minutes.

But what about more serious, longer-term effects? Most of the evidence suggests that drinking coffee doesn't increase the risk of cancer, and that tea contains ingredients (flavonoids and phenols) that may even have some protective effect against cancer, heart disease, and stroke. There's also some evidence that men who drink two or three cups of coffee a day have a 40 per cent lower risk of gallstones than men who don't drink it regularly. The only significant health risk could come from Scandinavian-style boiled coffee and coffee made in a 'cafetière'— these can increase cholesterol levels and the risk of heart disease, so it's best to drink them in moderation.

Overall, you should aim to restrict yourself to about 300 mg of caffeine a day, equivalent to about one pint of percolated ground coffee or almost two pints of tea.

WHAT'S IN YOUR CUPPA?

Drink	Caffeine (mg)
Instant coffee	66
Percolated ground coffee	74
Filter coffee	112
Espresso (30 ml cup)	75–115
Leaf tea	41
Tea bag	42
Instant tea	28
Cocoa drink	4
Cola (330 ml)	43–65

Average caffeine content in a 150 ml or 0.25 pint cup (unless specified)
Caffeine is also found in chocolate (20 mg in a 4 oz bar of milk chocolate and four times as much in dark), and in many pain killers and cold-relief products.

What's stopping you?

I love junk food—how can I give it up?

You don't have to stop eating junk food altogether—it's far more important to eat it at a level that's consistent with a generally healthy diet. Junk food's by no means identical, either: a fishcake is lower in fat and calories than a piece of battered fish, for example, while thick-cut fries absorb less fat than the thin-cut variety. Spice up pizzas with garlic and chilli rather than fatty pepperoni. If you prefer burgers, better choices include a plain burger or a cheeseburger (both without fries), and grab a diet cola rather than the milk-shake. Choose plain rice rather than Indian pilau rice or Chinese special fried rice, and if you want a kebab, go for a shish rather than a doner: it's got real, grilled meat and is served with salad and pitta bread.

I don't like fruit

How many sorts have you tried? Aside from the basics—apples, pears, oranges, and bananas—it's not hard now to get hold of kiwis, pineapples, mangoes, apricots, guavas, and papayas. Don't write off fruit until you've tried the lot. If you still hate it, try fruit juices or even dried fruit such as raisins, apricots, and prunes.

Salads are okay for rabbits but I need my meat and veg

Okay, so 'real' men don't eat quiche—or salad. And they don't need to: as long as

BETWEEN SEVEN STOOLS

Here's a new way to check the quality of your diet. Simply compare your stools with what doctors have dubbed 'The Bristol Scale'.

Stool type	Description
1	Separate hard lumps, like nuts.
2	Sausage-shaped but lumpy
3	Like a sausage or snake but with cracks on its surface
4	Like a sausage or snake, smooth and soft
5	Soft blobs with clear-cut edges
6	Fluffy pieces with ragged edges and mushy
7	Watery, no solid pieces

The perfect droppings are either type 3 or 4. If yours are in the lower numbers on the scale, try eating more wholemeal bread, bran flakes, and fruit; if they're in the higher numbers, cut down on these foods, as well as anything spicy and rich. Whatever your problem, drinking more water could also help.

If you have persistent constipation, blood in your stools or diarrhea that lasts for more than 48 hours, get medical advice.

you're eating enough vegetables, it doesn't matter too much whether they're cooked or raw. If you do boil vegetables, however, minimize the loss of important nutrients such as vitamin C by using only one inch of water, boiling it before adding the veg and never adding salt (it draws out the nutrients).

I don't want to become a vegetarian

You don't have to, at least not on health grounds. Although vegetarians tend to live longer than non-vegetarians, this is probably because they eat loads of fruit and vegetables. If you do the same, you can also safely eat limited amounts of meat.

I follow a healthy diet but I just can't stop farting

A diet containing lots of relatively indigestible foods like beans, Brussels sprouts, onions, peas, or added bran can cause a problem with bottom burps. Try reducing your intake of these sorts of foods until the problem is under control (note that 21 farts a day is considered normal) and then slowly increasing it again. Drinking more water, eating live yoghurt, and drinking peppermint tea after meals might also help. Your problem could also be exacerbated if you eat foods sweetened with sorbitol (it's widely used in ready-made desserts, and vast amounts of gas are produced as it ferments in the gut) or your digestive system can't handle lactose (the natural sugar in milk). Cut these out in turn and see if you notice a difference.

Food for fitness

Unless you're an elite athlete or a bodybuilder who needs a very carefully controlled diet, the odds are that you'll perform perfectly well on a normal, healthy diet that is generally high in carbohydrate and low in fat. It's carbohydrate, stored in the muscles as glycogen, that forms the key fuel for exercise.

Key tips:

➲ Don't exercise within three to four hours of eating a large meal or within two to three hours of a medium meal—give your stomach time to empty or you could feel bloated and uncomfortable. But a small, high-carbohydrate snack within 30 minutes of exercise can improve your performance (try a large banana or a low-fat cereal bar).

➲ Drink water generously in the two hours before exercise to help prevent dehydration. During exercise, sip some fluid (water or diluted fruit juice) regularly, especially if you're in a hot environment.

➲ After exercise, rehydrate your body—again with water or diluted fruit juice.

➲ Don't waste your money on special sports supplements. Sports drinks can provide fast fluid replacement and fight dehydration and fatigue, but for most of us plain water will do fine. (The only exception might be for a high-intensity endurance event lasting longer than 90 minutes, like marathon running, when a drink containing a small amount of glucose could improve stamina.)

➲ Don't drink alcohol straight after exercise—it will dehydrate you further. If you do fancy some booze, drink water or juice first.

➲ Restore glycogen levels by eating some carbohydrate within two hours of exercise; it doesn't need to be a sports snack bar either—a banana sandwich or just a lump of bread will do and cost you less.

➲ Forget about taking extra vitamins and minerals. Although it's often claimed they boost muscular strength and endurance, speed up post-exercise recovery, prevent injury, and increase aerobic capacity, there's actually no good evidence that supplementation has any effect on sports performance. Protein supplements are also unnecessary and sometimes an outright con—

researchers found that one leading protein drink actually provided less protein than a normal serving of roasted chicken breast or tuna. Most sportsmen can do perfectly well on the amounts found in a normal, healthy diet.

THINGS YOU DIDN'T KNOW ABOUT FOOD

○ Life is sweet. If you think eating confectionery must be bad for you, you're wrong. A study of over 7800 American men found that, on average, men who ate candy live almost a year longer than abstainers. Those who indulged one to three times a month live longest. The study didn't differentiate between chocolate and sugar candy, but the researchers speculated that chocolate could be the key factor: it contains antioxidants, which could lower the risk of heart disease and cancer.

○ Go nuts. Eating nuts five or more times a week could reduce your risk of heart disease by 35 per cent compared to non or infrequent nut eaters, according to a recent large-scale study. Other research suggests the reduced risk might even be as high as 50 per cent. Although nuts are high in fat, the fat is mostly unsaturated; this can help reduce cholesterol levels. Nuts also contain magnesium, vitamin E, fiber, and potassium, ingredients known to protect against heart disease. But don't go mad: nuts are very calorie-dense, and a total of just five ounces a week could be enough to make a difference.

○ High-fat foods could make you drowsy because of cholecystokinin (CCK), a substance released in the duodenum in response to fat. Research at the Centre for Human Nutrition at Sheffield University in the UK has shown that when CCK is given intravenously to volunteers, they experience the same drowsiness and decline in performance that follows the consumption of high-fat foods. It's no coincidence that most celebratory meals are replete with a variety of high-fat foods and that almost everyone falls asleep during the after-dinner speeches.

○ Whatever you eat, it's difficult to counter the effects of the post-lunch dip. (This is largely due to the body's internal clock.) But its effects can be reduced by keeping your lunches small: work requiring accuracy is affected more by a heavy lunch (about 1000 calories) than a light lunch (300 calories); moreover, if you eat a larger meal than normal, you may well experience greater performance impairments than if you eat a smaller meal than usual. A cup of coffee can also help early afternoon concentration, increasing the speed of rapid information processing by about 10 per cent.

CHAPTER 7

FIXING THE FIX:
HOW TO UNHOOK YOUR ADDICTIONS

We probably don't want to admit it, even to ourselves, but most of us are addicted to something. Millions of men have stopped smoking, but over a quarter of us are still hooked. Alcohol is commonly consumed above safe levels, and drugs such as cannabis, cocaine, and heroin are widely used despite being illegal. Although their effects aren't nearly so serious, it's even possible to develop a seemingly uncontrollable craving for caffeine, chocolate, or sugar. But not all addictions involve chemical substances. Compulsive gambling is a well-known problem, and in the last few years, psychologists have identified addictions to work, sex, pornography, and even the Internet. It's almost no exaggeration to say that we live in an addicted society, one in which addictive behavior is the norm rather than the exception.

Although both men and women are affected, men are generally more likely to become hooked. Perhaps it's because we're more willing to take risks or because we'd rather deal with personal problems by distracting ourselves with an addiction than talking them through with a partner or friend. Some addictions have become so much part of everyday male culture that we've grown up believing that activities like drinking too much or working all hours are actually completely normal. One particular irony for men is that, although we like to feel in total control of our lives, an addiction can eventually take control of us. But it doesn't have to be like this: we can get off the hook and, by doing so, provide the best possible shot in the arm for our physical and mental health.

STUB OUT SMOKING FOR GOOD

The male hall of fame is clogged with smokers. Every day, James Bond puffs his way through 70 high-tar, unfiltered cigarettes made from a blend of black Turkish tobaccos. In the classic film *Casablanca*, night-club proprietor Rick Blaine (Humphrey Bogart) effortlessly outwits the Nazis while permanently enveloped in a cloud of his own cigarette fumes. These men aren't worried about developing a cough, let alone cancer. They behave as if their lungs were made of titanium and their hearts of reinforced concrete, so little concern do they show about the health risks they are so obviously running.

But their essential organs, like everyone's, are actually made of soft and vulnerable tissues that don't take kindly to nicotine or the hundreds of other toxic ingredients stuffed inside a cigarette. Humphrey Bogart died of cancer of the esophagus, a disease often caused by smoking. If he really existed, James Bond almost certainly would have developed lung cancer (that's if the booze, sexually transmitted infections, or stray bullets hadn't got him first). About half of all regular cigarette smokers will eventually be killed by their habit; on average, every time a smoker lights up, he's shortening his life by more than five minutes. Giving up smoking may mean giving up part of the image we have of ourselves as men—fast-living, carefree, risk-taking, rebellious, even heroic—but the gains surely outweigh the losses: a longer life, firmer erections, a higher sperm count, and breath that no longer smells like an ashtray.

Why bother to quit smoking?

○ Twenty minutes after quitting, your blood pressure and pulse rate return to normal. Circulation improves in the hands and feet, making them warmer.
○ After eight hours, oxygen levels in the blood return to normal and the chances of a heart attack start to fall.
○ Sleep improves on the first night after quitting as nicotine levels are reduced. One study of very heavy smokers (40 a day) found that the time taken to fall asleep fell from 52 to 18 minutes.
○ After 24 hours, carbon monoxide is eliminated from the body. The lungs start to clear out mucus and other debris.
○ 48 hours after your last cigarette, nicotine is no longer detectable in the body. Your ability to taste and smell improves, and you will also begin to smell and taste better to others.
○ After 72 hours, breathing becomes easier as the bronchial tubes relax. Your energy levels will increase.
○ Between two and twelve weeks after giving up, circulation improves throughout the body. Your erections should become firmer and longer-lasting. Over a longer period, your overall penis length could also begin to increase slightly, and you're much less likely to develop erectile dysfunction (impotence)— smoking is implicated in up to 80 per cent of cases of erection problems.

○ After three to nine months, breathing problems such as cough, shortness of breath, and wheezing improve. Overall lung function is up 5–10 per cent. Since smokers' sperm concentrations are on average some 15 per cent lower than those of non-smokers, quitting could also produce a significant increase in the quality of your semen.

○ One year after quitting, the increased risk of coronary heart disease you faced as a smoker has halved. After 15 years, the risk is similar to that of someone who has never smoked.

○ The risk of developing lung cancer falls. One study found that stopping smoking after 30 years reduces the risk of death from this disease by about 80 per cent over the next 15 years.

○ If you're a smoker, quitting is probably the single most important step you can take to improve your health and prolong your life. You'll also save an enormous amount of money.

I'm puffed out—how can I change?

○ Be clear about your motivation. Is it because of worries about your health or perhaps the health of your children? Are cigarettes costing you too much? Are you fed up with feeling like a second-class citizen because you're not allowed to smoke at work or in an increasing number of other public places?

○ Make a definite commitment. Set a date and time for giving up and stick to it. But be realistic, too: don't try it the day before you've got a job interview or if your dog's just died.

○ Keep a 'smoking diary'. Noting down when you light up and what's happening at the time could help you identify your key smoking triggers. For example, you may find that you have a cigarette after a meal or every time you have to make a difficult telephone call at work. This will make you aware of when you particularly need to be on your guard and to work out alternatives to having a puff. Perhaps a cup of tea, or walking up and down two flights of stairs, would make a difference.

○ Go for broke—in other words, complete abstinence. Don't try a gradual reduction approach: the evidence is that it doesn't work because it saps the will to stop—the more you cut down, the more important each remaining cigarette becomes and the harder it is to give up the last few.

○ Forget about aversion therapy, such as smoking 50 cigarettes one after the other to get a nicotine overdose. Even if the nausea, vomiting, dizziness, and palpitations did create a long-lasting aversion, the technique is too hazardous to be worth considering seriously.

THE SCIENCE BIT

○ Smokers look older. One study of 268 British men found that smokers are twice as likely to be balding than non-smokers and over four times as likely to have grey hair. Smoking is also associated with premature facial wrinkles. It was possible for doctors in one study to identify about half of those who had smoked for 10 years or more by their facial features alone.

○ Smoking causes cancer. Almost nine out of ten cases of lung cancer in men are caused by smoking. According to a study of over 34,000 British male doctors, if you smoke 1–14 cigarettes a day, your risk of developing the disease is eight times that of a non-smoker; if you smoke 15–24, your risk rises to 15 times; if you smoke 25 or more, it's 25 times greater. Smoking also increases the risk of cancers of the mouth, throat, bladder, kidney, and pancreas.

○ Even light cigarette smoking increases the risk of heart disease, according to a study of almost 7000 middle-aged Swedish men. Men who smoke just one to four cigarettes a day are three times more likely to develop it.

○ Smokers in their 30s and 40s have five times as many heart attacks as non-smokers, according to a study of 10,000 UK heart attack survivors. In fact, when a smoker of this age has a heart attack, there's an 80 per cent chance tobacco caused it.

○ Smokers are more likely to suffer from minor health complaints than non-smokers. A UK survey found that smokers reported 60 per cent more symptoms of problems like colds, flu, fatigue, earache, toothache, and eyestrain.

○ Your smoking can harm others. Fifteen per cent of childhood cancers are linked to smoking by fathers, according to an analysis of the smoking habits of the parents of over 1500 children who died of cancer in the UK. There's also a 10–30 per cent increased risk of lung cancer in non-smokers who've experienced a lifetime's exposure to environmental tobacco smoke.

○ Chuck out all your smoking materials and paraphernalia (lighters, ashtrays, etc.). This should make it harder for you to start smoking again if your determination temporarily weakens.

○ In the early days it might help to avoid situations where you might be tempted to smoke. This could mean, for example, not going out for a drink with colleagues at lunchtime or straight after work.

○ Try to quit with others. You can provide mutual encouragement and share how bad you feel with people who really understand what you're going through. It's also worth making use of the expert advice and support you can access through quitters' groups.

○ Ease the withdrawal symptoms with nicotine-replacement therapies (NRTs)— the research shows that the patches, gum, inhaler, or nasal spray all double the chances of success. But don't expect any NRT to be a magic cure: all it can do is reduce the cravings for a cigarette, not make them go away. Nevertheless, it should reduce withdrawal symptoms and it's certainly better than going cold turkey. There's also emerging evidence that the anti-depressant drug bupropion (marketed as Zyban) can help quitting, either in combination with an NRT or on its own.

○ Consider acupuncture. Although the evidence of its effectiveness is mixed, one careful study found definite benefits from an intensive program (acupuncture six times in three weeks plus self-help 'acupressure' four times daily). Practitioners normally work with acupoints on the ear.

○ Consider meditation. Several studies have found that over half of smokers who consistently meditate are more likely than non-meditators or irregular meditators to quit. One plausible theory is that meditation works because it reduces anxiety.

○ Don't be discouraged by a relapse. Rather than feeling guilty or a failure, focus on what you've already achieved and think about how you can make your next attempt even more effective.

What's stopping you?

Smoking helps me concentrate
It's true—nicotine improves the transmission of nerve impulses in the hippocampus, the part of the brain involved in learning and memory. But does this advantage outweigh the dangers?

Cigarettes relieve my stress
No they don't—all they relieve is the withdrawal symptoms you experience since your last smoke. This explains why, after smokers have quit and got through the withdrawal period, they actually experience reduced levels of daily stress.

I don't like the withdrawal symptoms
You're not alone—they're enough to keep almost anyone hooked. You can expect to feel hungry, tired, irritable, depressed, and light-headed—as well as desperate

---

QUITTERS: THE FACTS

- Over half of all smokers want to stop and one in six are actually trying to do so at any one time.
- Over half of those who want to stop want to do so for health reasons and almost 40 per cent want to quit because of the cost.
- The most common trigger for stopping is something said by a family member or friend.
- Almost half of quitters don't use any particular method, relying solely on will-power.
- Although most smokers have to try to quit several times, around half eventually succeed.

---

for a cigarette. And this will last two to four weeks. The good news is that there are ways of reducing their impact, especially through nicotine-replacement therapies.

It helps keep my weight down

Smoking does suppress the appetite, and each cigarette stimulates the body to burn up eight extra calories. Men gain an average of about six pounds when they quit smoking, but this amount can easily be lost once smoking withdrawal has been successfully dealt with.

I'll switch to low-tar smokes

It's hardly worth it—the smoke from low-tar cigarettes tends to be inhaled more deeply because it's less irritating to the airways, causing a build-up of tar and, potentially, tumors deeper in the lungs. Switching from a high-tar to a low-tar brand might make you feel virtuous but its effect on your health will be negligible. There's no longer any doubt: the only good cigarette is a stubbed-out cigarette.

OK, I'll try cigars instead

Once again, any advantage will be marginal. A single cigar can contain as much tobacco as a whole pack of cigarettes and, although cigar smokers tend not to inhale directly, they're still breathing in the smoke swirling in the air around them. A large study of US men aged 30–85 who'd never smoked cigarettes found that cigar smokers are 27 per cent more likely to develop heart disease compared to non-smokers and over twice as likely to suffer from lung cancer.

My grandfather smoked 30 a day and lived to be 95
He was lucky—and there'll always be some men who are. But it's more important to look at the overall statistics rather than isolated cases. A study of over 7700 British men concluded that only 42 per cent of lifelong smokers would still be alive at the age of 73 compared with 78 per cent of lifelong non-smokers. In other words, smokers are almost twice as likely to die before they reach their early 70s.

THINGS YOU DIDN'T KNOW ABOUT SMOKING

○ Smoking delivers nicotine to the brain faster than an intravenous injection—the first puffs of a cigarette produce a near immediate 'hit' or 'buzz', a feeling of intoxication and excitement. In fact, nicotine stimulates the same area of the brain—the 'central reward pathway'—that is affected by heroin and cocaine.

○ Becoming a dad could help you quit. An analysis of 16,000 16–49-year-olds in the UK found that men with two or more children were 25 per cent more likely to stop smoking than childless men. Explanations could include concern about children's health, a desire to prevent children taking up the habit, and direct nagging from children themselves.

○ Smokers used to be able to claim that, for all its faults, their habit at least protected them against Alzheimer's disease. But the latest research has reversed previous medical thinking. A Dutch study of 6870 people aged 55 years and over found that smoking was actually associated with a doubling of the risk of Alzheimer's.

○ Passive smoking can also affect pets. A US study of over 100 dogs with nasal cancer found the risks to man's best friends significantly increase when they live with a smoker. Long-nosed dogs are at particularly high risk.

○ Smoking's even bad for the environment. A modern cigarette-manufacturing machine uses four miles of paper per hour, cigarette ends take up to two years to degrade naturally, and it's been estimated that, world-wide, smoking generates about 2.6 billion kg of carbon monoxide and 5.2 billion kg of methane every year—these are gases responsible for the greenhouse effect.

○ Smokers' efforts to quit are being undermined by a rise in smoking in the movies, according to University of California research. In films from the 1970s and 1980s, smoking occurred once every 10–15 minutes on average. But in the 1990s, it took place every three to five minutes.

Some good news at last. Once men make up their minds to quit, research suggests they're more likely to succeed than women.

WIN THE BATTLE OF THE BOTTLE

If you've ever felt embarrassed walking up to a bar and ordering an orange juice or a mineral water then it's probably because you know that, however good they might taste, soft drinks simply aren't 'men's drinks'. As we all know, men are supposed to drink the 'hard stuff'—and the more they can put away, the more of a man they are. This wouldn't matter much if alcohol had the same effect on the body as orange juice or mineral water. When consumed in man-size quantities, however, alcohol is rather more hazardous.

But not all alcohol is dangerous: you probably don't have to stop drinking to enjoy a healthy relationship with drink—in fact, some alcohol might actually be good for you, and none of that watery alcohol-free beer need ever pass your lips (unless you want it to, of course).

Why bother to control your drinking?

○ No more hangovers.
○ You'll sleep better. While one or two drinks might help you sleep, more tends to affect both sleep quality and quantity, leaving you feeling groggier than normal in the mornings.
○ You could lose weight. Alcohol not only increases your calorie intake and can contribute to weight gain, it also erodes your ability to resist fattening foods like peanuts, burgers, and fries.
○ Your sexual desire could increase. Large amounts of alcohol can inhibit the body's production of testosterone, the key hormone regulating your libido.
○ You'll perform better sexually. Too much alcohol can reduce your pleasure as well as that of your partner. Alcohol-laden belches are also not likely to go down too well with your partner.
○ You'll be a lot healthier. Regular heavy boozing is associated with such stomach problems as gastritis as well as cirrhosis of the liver, diabetes, hepatitis, and several cancers.

What's a safe level of drinking?

Different experts give different advice, but the bulk of the evidence suggests you'd be sensible to set a limit of no more than 21 units a week. Your daily maximum should be three or four units a day, and you should aim for one or two drink-free days each week. You're at increasing risk of an alcohol-related health problem if you regularly drink more than four units a day.

1 unit of alcohol = 8 grams or 10 ml of alcohol =
- ○ 0.5 pints (284 ml or 10 fluid ounces) of ordinary beer, lager, or cider.
- ○ 1 single measure (25 ml or one-sixth of a gill) of spirits (whisky, gin, rum, vodka, etc.).
- ○ 1 small glass (95 ml or 3 fluid ounces) of wine.

The 'standard' US drinks of 340 ml of beer, 42.6 ml of spirits, and 132 ml of wine are equivalent to 1.2, 1.7, and 1.4 units respectively.

Can alcohol really be good for you?

Evidence is mounting that light or moderate drinkers are less likely to die of heart disease than both non-drinkers and heavy drinkers. A study of over 12,000 British doctors found that those drinking 8–14 units a week had the lowest risk of dying. The most beneficial level of consumption is thought to be one or two drinks a day consumed over five or six days a week—knocking back the same total amount each week in fewer drinking sessions just doesn't have the same effect. To be sure of getting any of these benefits, you should stick to red wine—it's particularly rich in antioxidants and flavonoids, substances believed to have a role in reducing heart disease—although some research suggests that any type of alcohol produces similar results. But—and it's a big but—the benefits of alcohol start only when the risks of heart disease become significant; for men, that's after the age of about 40. Younger men can't seriously claim they're hanging out in bars to protect their hearts.

Alcohol doesn't just reduce the risk of heart disease, however. There's also some evidence that drinking up to five units a day can reduce the risk of gallstones, while drinking nine units or more of alcohol a week can significantly reduce the risk of being infected with *Helicobacter pylori*, a bacterium known to cause peptic ulcers.

I'm fed up with hangovers—how can I change?

- ○ Be clear about why you want to change. Do you want to lose weight, for example? Do you want to improve your fitness or your sports performance? Is your drinking causing problems in your relationship or with work? Are you spending too much money on alcohol? Are you worried about how it affects your behavior (e.g. because you become abusive or even violent)? Are you experiencing memory black-outs after binge-drinking sessions?
- ○ Commit yourself to making the change. This is important, because adopting a new relationship with alcohol won't necessarily be easy. If you started drinking

THE SCIENCE BIT

○ Alcohol causes accidents. If your blood contains 50 mg of alcohol per 100 ml of blood, your chances of having a road accident are doubled; at 80 mg, the risk increases fourfold; at 160 mg, the chances of an accident are 50 times higher. Two to three units (see opposite) can be enough to push alcohol blood levels up to 50 mg. Heavy drinking is also associated with deaths by drowning, domestic accidents, and a large proportion of deaths in fires.

○ Booze increases the risk of certain cancers. There may be as much as a 20-fold increase in the risk of cancer of the esophagus (or gullet) and a significantly increased risk of cancers of the mouth and throat, according to a review of all the evidence by the World Cancer Research Fund. The risk of these cancers starts to increase if you drink four to five units a day, although regular heavy drinkers are at greatest risk. There's also convincing evidence that alcohol can contribute to liver cancer and that it's linked to cancers of the colon and rectum.

○ High levels of drinking are associated with raised blood pressure which, in turn, is a significant risk factor for coronary heart disease and stroke. One in 10 cases of high blood pressure is thought to be caused primarily by alcohol.

○ Alcohol can cause sexual problems. Tests on men shown erotic movies suggest that even moderate amounts of alcohol slow the body's physical response during sexual arousal—basically, men take longer to achieve an erection. A study of male alcohol addicts in New Zealand found that almost three quarters had suffered from a sexual dysfunction for at least 12 months.

○ Alcohol affects physical fitness by damaging muscle fibers. In the short term, it reduces stamina, compromising performance—for instance, in the second half of a football match. In the long-term, the muscle fibers necessary for short sprints and jumping are damaged. Long-term alcohol misuse can affect more than fitness, however: up to 20 per cent of the entire skeletal musculature can be lost.

○ Binge drinking can be particularly dangerous. A Finnish study of over 1600 middle-aged male beer drinkers found that those consuming six or more bottles per session were three times more likely to die within about 10 years than those who usually drank a maximum of three bottles per session. The binge drinkers were six times more likely to suffer a fatal heart attack.

heavily to deal with anxiety or depression, for example, you could find that once you reduce or stop your drinking you'll start to feel all the unpleasant feelings once again. Alternatively, you might face the problem that many or all of your social relationships now revolve around drinking; cutting back could therefore have major implications for your social life.

○ Work out exactly how much you're drinking now. The best way to do this is to start a 'drink diary'—each day, write down what you drank the day before (e.g. '5 pints of beer—10 units') as well as when and where you drank and with whom. Add how you were feeling just before you started drinking—were you angry or tense, for example? You must be completely honest with yourself—include the one-off lunchtime drinks, and allow for the larger measures you probably pour yourself at home. At the end of the week, total up the number of units.

○ If you're drinking more than 21 units a week, analyze the circumstances in which you're drinking excessively. Is it with colleagues after work? Is it at lunchtime? Is it with a particular group of friends? Is it when you're feeling tense or upset? This could help you avoid those situations in which you tend to drink too much and think about other ways of coping with uncomfortable feelings like anxiety, anger, stress, loneliness, or guilt. Talking to your partner, a friend, or a counselor might help. Taking regular aerobic exercise and practicing simple relaxation techniques such as slow, deep breathing could also make a difference.

○ Decide whether you should cut down or stop drinking completely. Abstinence can be harder to achieve, but could be a better long-term option if you're currently a very heavy drinker. In fact, if you're drinking at a level where you experience severe withdrawal symptoms—such as restlessness, agitation, trembling, nausea, and sleeplessness—your best bet is to see a doctor or a specialist counselor before you try to cut back.

○ If you choose to carry on drinking, try setting yourself a limit each time you drink. If you decide in advance that you'll drink no more than, say, two pints of beer in an evening, you're more likely to stick to it than if you drink two pints and then attempt to think about when you stop.

○ Pace yourself when you drink to try to establish the habit of drinking more slowly. You could also try switching to smaller or less alcoholic drinks (e.g. half pints rather than pints, regular lager instead of premium or extra strong), alternating alcoholic and non-alcoholic drinks, or missing the occasional round. If you drink with food you'll probably drink less—and more slowly.

○ Get support. Whether you're giving up alcohol or cutting down, you'll probably find it easier if you can share the experience with others. Perhaps you and your partner (or a friend) could decide to help each other. You might even create a financial incentive by agreeing that whoever starts drinking too much first has to make a substantial donation to charity. If you're a heavier drinker, a group like Alcoholics' Anonymous could prove more useful.

○ There's evidence that acupuncture can ease alcohol withdrawal symptoms and that people who meditate regularly are much more likely than non-meditators to stop or reduce their drinking.

What's stopping you?

I like the taste of alcohol

Yep, there's nothing quite like it—and certainly not those so-called 'beers' and 'wines' sold as alcohol-free. But remember, the first drink always tastes best—the more you drink (and the more numb your brain becomes), the less well you can taste. If you sip your drink rather than take large gulps, you'll not only be able to savor the taste but also drink more slowly.

It's an important part of my social life

It still can be, even if you start drinking less.

Key tips:

➲ If you're going out with friends and you're not going to drink, you could offer to be the driver.

➲ Suggest that you try some new activities that aren't focused on drinking (e.g. ten-pin bowling or going out for a meal).

➲ Accept that your relationships might be affected if you start drinking less. It'll help if you tell your friends that you've decided to cut back and explain why. But a few of your friends might think you've become a wimp and you could start to get bored with some of their drunken antics. You may decide that 21st-century Man doesn't need to prove his masculinity by getting drunk and being sick in the bath.

➲ Be open to new friendships with people who aren't so interested in alcohol.

A few drinks help me relax and deal with stress

This isn't a good long-term strategy because alcohol can't tackle the causes of your stress—at best, it can temporarily relieve the symptoms. But there's also a danger that as you get into the habit of drinking to relax, you'll need more to achieve the same effect. In time, you could actually be drinking more to prevent withdrawal symptoms than to relieve your stress—and the underlying causes of stress will still be there.

HANGOVERS

Hangovers are caused by a combination of dehydration, the effects of toxic substances in alcohol called congeners, and interrupted sleep due to alcohol withdrawal during the night. Hangovers can affect your attention and concentration for up to 16 hours after you've finished drinking, even if you feel sober.

FIVE WAYS TO AVOID A HANGOVER

○ Drink water—as much as you can before, during, and after alcohol. It'll help you avoid dehydration.

○ Start eating before you start imbibing—it'll help delay the absorption of alcohol. At the very least, drink some milk or eat something fatty, but unsalted—salty food will increase your thirst; plain almonds are a good bet.

○ From your brain cells' point of view, the lower the alcohol concentration the better, making beer just about the best choice. If you prefer spirits, consider iced vodka. Vodka is free of congeners, and cold drinks tend to be absorbed more slowly than those at room temperature.

○ Avoid darker-colored alcohol (e.g. whisky, brandy, sherry, or red wine)—it's stuffed with congeners. And avoid all fizzy concoctions: they're potential time-bombs, because carbon dioxide speeds up alcohol absorption into the blood.

○ A final option—just don't drink too much.

FIVE WAYS TO CURE A HANGOVER

○ Lie in bed, drink a lot (that means water, sweet tea, or diluted fruit juice) and take some paracetemol. Avoid aspirin—it can irritate the stomach lining.

○ Apply an ice-pack: 20 minutes on and 10 minutes off can help ease the throbbing.

○ Try *Nux vomica*. This homeopathic remedy is particularly recommended if you also feel cold, irritable, and over-sensitive to noise.

○ If you can, eat carbohydrate-rich foods (plain bread or toast, cereal, fruit) and steer clear of fatty fry-ups and croissants. You need stuff your stomach can handle without doing overtime.

○ Fancy a traditional remedy? Witchcraft lore recommends driving a nail into a wax effigy of someone you don't like in order to transfer the hangover to them. It's worth a try if you're desperate.

I can handle my liquor

People do have different tolerances for alcohol: generally, the larger and heavier you are the more slowly your blood alcohol level will rise, and if you're a regular heavy drinker, your liver will metabolize alcohol faster while nerve cells in your brain will be less responsive to its effects. But these are all warning signs: being overweight is a health risk in its own right, and changes in your liver and brain that enable you to tolerate more alcohol suggest that you might actually be addicted. If you're being honest, are you really in control?

THINGS YOU DIDN'T KNOW ABOUT ALCOHOL

- All of us, drinkers or not, have some alcohol in our blood all the time. It's produced as a result of the action of digestive juices on the sugars and starches we eat.
- Alcohol significantly speeds up the passage of food from the mouth through the gut to the anus. One study found average 'transit' times are 49 hours for men drinking over five units a day but 54 hours for those drinking under 2.5 units a day.
- Men are generally able to digest alcohol more quickly than women because their stomachs contain higher levels of an alcohol-eliminating enzyme known as alcohol dehydrogenase (ADH). This means that, drink-for-drink, less alcohol gets into a man's bloodstream from his stomach, enabling him to tolerate more alcohol than a woman.

COMPULSIONS AREN'T COMPULSORY

What about other addictions? What warning signs do we need to look out for and what can we do if we spot them?

What's your poison?

- **Sex**. Some men find that sex has become compulsive. Such a compulsion often involves having lots of partners, anonymous sexual encounters, or a pursuit of sex despite a risk to other relationships, health, or employment. It's also possible to become hooked on pornography.

○ **The Internet**. Up to three per cent of Internet users could be seriously addicted, spending almost 40 hours a week online compared to an average of under five hours a week for non-dependent users.

○ **Exercise**. Some men can experience withdrawal symptoms if they're unable to work out. In one study of runners, just two weeks' abstinence produced a variety of health complaints, insomnia, and feelings of depression and anxiety.

○ **Drugs**. Illegal drugs are widely used: 45 per cent of 16–29-year-olds have taken drugs, according to one UK survey; cannabis is by far the most popular, tried by 36 per cent. One in 12 UK gym users admits to trying anabolic steroids.

○ **Gambling**. Compulsive gamblers are unable to resist an opportunity to experience the excitement of placing a bet and hoping for a big win.

○ **Caffeine**. Just four or five cups of ground coffee a day can be enough to cause unpleasant withdrawal symptoms if there's an attempt to cut down.

○ **Work**. As jobs become increasingly insecure, more men are turning into workaholics, regularly working more than 50 hours a week and having very few other interests.

○ **Shopping**. Seven per cent of men are now reckoned to be shopaholics, bingeing on clothes, shoes, compact discs, and tools.

○ *Star Trek*. A study of fans attending *Star Trek* conventions in the UK found that up to 15 per cent showed signs of a serious addiction: they watched the program to improve their mood and felt irritable when they couldn't get enough.

Are you really addicted?

Psychologists believe an activity can be described as an addiction when at least two or three of the following are present:

○ Salience. The activity has become the most important activity in your life and dominates your thinking, feelings, and behavior.
○ Euphoria. The activity produces a buzz or high. Sometimes, however, you may experience a tranquilizing or numbing feeling.

○ Tolerance. Increasing amounts of the activity are required to achieve euphoria.
○ Withdrawal symptoms. You experience unpleasant feelings (e.g. moodiness or irritability) when the activity is stopped or reduced.
○ Conflict. Your behavior causes conflict either with others or within your own mind.
○ Relapse. You can't stop the behavior despite your best efforts to do so.

I'm hooked—how can I change?

If you're addicted, and want to do something about it, it could help to follow a program that will identify the roots of your compulsion and enable you to take practical steps to change your behavior. If you are addicted to drugs, however, you almost certainly need to seek expert help. It may be necessary for you to take other drugs to minimize any withdrawal symptoms and/or receive psychological support to help tackle the problems that led to the drug use in the first place.

Key tips:
➲ Be motivated. You have to be sure why you want to end your addiction and you must be clear that it's for your own benefit, not to please others.
➲ Understand your triggers. Keep a careful written record of each time you gamble, use the Internet, etc. Beside each entry, note what you were doing and how you were feeling at the time. You might discover that your addiction is linked to feelings of stress or loneliness or being with people who share your addiction.
➲ Decide whether you're going to cut down or give up. This may depend on how severe your addiction is and whether it's safe for you to carry on with the behavior even on a controlled basis. If you opt for continuing, set yourself strict groundrules. If you break them more than a few times, consider complete abstinence.
➲ Find alternatives. If you've identified your addiction triggers, you can then try to develop satisfying non-addictive substitutes. If you find that you tend to gamble when you feel bored, frustrated, or angry, for example, you can decide to do something else instead when you recognize you have those feelings (e.g. have a bath, go for a walk, listen to music, try relaxation exercises).
➲ Examine your beliefs about your addiction. Addicts find all sorts of ways to justify their behavior to themselves. Gamblers are convinced their luck's about to change and that they'll soon have a big win, for instance, while sex addicts believe another conquest will make them feel powerful and attractive. Are your justifications rational?

➲ Learn to deal with relapses. A relapse doesn't mean you might as well give up. It's far better to see it as a learning opportunity: look at what happened, try and work out why, and devise strategies to prevent it occurring again.

➲ Get support. Being able to talk about what's going on and getting the encouragement of others is crucial. Try a partner, friends, family, a counselor, or a support group like Gamblers or Sex Addicts Anonymous.

Giving up any addiction is tough work, but ultimately satisfying and rewarding. Not only will you be emotionally and physically healthier but you will also gain some valuable insights into your psyche. Most importantly, you will have achieved a sense of control over your life. You will be the one in charge, not your addiction.

CHAPTER 8

DEAD TIRED?
ENJOY THE REST OF YOUR LIFE

You've decided to have an early night and have just dropped off to sleep when the phone rings. On hearing your groggy answer, the caller asks if you were asleep. Needless to say, you vehemently deny it. Partly you don't want the caller to feel guilty; but a much bigger factor is that you'd feel embarrassed, even ashamed, to admit to being asleep by 10pm. Even if you're exhausted, crashing out much before midnight seems boring and, above all, distinctly unmanly. The only time 'real' men hit the sack is when they're too drunk to stand, have been fatally wounded in battle, or want to spend the next eight hours enjoying the kind of sex most of us can only fantasize about.

What's more, the development of the fast-paced, high-tech, 24-hour society means that more and more of us aren't getting enough shut-eye. Sixty-two per cent of the British population get fewer hours of sleep than five years ago and increasingly use weekends and holidays to catch up on lost sleep, according to research by the UK Sleep Council. A US National Sleep Foundation survey found that 40 per cent of adults say they're so sleepy that it interferes with their daily activities, and 62 per cent experience problems sleeping for at least a few nights a week. If the only consequence was that too little sleep made us feel tired then the problem might not be so bad, but there's now increasing evidence that sleep deprivation can affect our physical and emotional health. We actually need sleep as much as we need healthy food and plenty of exercise.

Why bother about sleep?

○ If you sleep for as long as you need, the chances are you'll feel much better. You don't need to be a sleep scientist to know that you're more likely to feel good and perform well after a good night's shut-eye.

REAL HEALTH FOR MEN

○ Your immune system is likely to be stronger, increasing your resistance to a range of diseases from the common cold to more serious problems.
○ You'll be at much less risk of causing a road accident—all you'll have to do is avoid the other drivers whose eyelids are propped open with matchsticks.
○ You'll enjoy a better social life. There's good evidence that people who sleep well have better quality social interactions the following day.
○ If you feel rested and refreshed the odds are you'll feel more positive and optimistic, experience less stress, consume a better diet (less chocolate or caffeine will be needed for energy boosts), feel more like exercising, and be more motivated to participate in cultural activities. You might well want to have more sex, too—and be less inclined to fall asleep immediately afterwards. Combine all this with the direct benefits of sleep itself and you've accumulated some serious health advantages.

Do you have a sleep problem?

There's no need to worry if you don't sleep for exactly eight hours. The idea that we all need this amount every night is simply a myth. All we really need is enough to enable us to do what we need to do without feeling tired; for most of us, that's somewhere between six and nine hours a night. But what's even more important than the quantity of sleep is its quality: research suggests that you could well feel rougher after seven hours' sleep that's interrupted by two or three short awakenings than after six hours of solid sleep. It also pays to fall asleep reasonably quickly: for many of us, it's an even better predictor of feeling in a good mood the following day than the total length of sleep.

You could have a sleep problem if one or more of the following statements applies to you:
○ I fall asleep the minute my head hits the pillow.
○ I use medication or alcohol to help me sleep.
○ I usually take more than 30 minutes to fall asleep, either at the beginning of the night or if I wake up during the night.
○ I often wake up earlier than I'd like and can't get back to sleep.
○ My sleep is usually less restorative and refreshing than I'd like.
○ I often feel sleepy during the day.
○ I usually have to try to keep myself awake or alert by moving around, turning the heating down, drinking coffee, etc.
○ At weekends I need to sleep in late or nap to make up for lost sleep during the week.

THE SCIENCE BIT

○ Sleep problems are associated with poorer health and a reduced quality of life, according to a survey of almost 600 employees at a San Francisco Bay Area telecommunications company. The poor sleepers reported lower levels of energy, poorer mental functioning, decreased job performance, and worse general health than colleagues who didn't experience problems.

○ Laboratory studies indicate that losing as little as 80 minutes' sleep for one night can result in a reduction of daytime alertness by as much as 32 per cent. On a scale of one to 100 for overall functioning, sleep-deprived people score nine while the average well-rested person scores 50.

○ Weight-lifters who were limited by researchers to three hours of sleep a night for three days performed less well on three out of four exercises after the second night, suggesting that lack of sleep leads to increased muscle weakness. Another study of men who were deprived of sleep for 48 hours detected a significant decline in their ability to perform six different physical tasks involving all the major muscle groups.

○ Up to one-fifth of vehicle accidents are sleep-related, according to one study of accidents on major UK roads. The US National Highway Traffic Safety Administration reckons drowsy driving causes at least 100,000 crashes a year.

○ Four hours' sleep deprivation causes an immediate 28 per cent fall in immune-system functioning, according to a study of healthy men aged 22–61. After a night's normal sleep, immune activity returns to normal levels.

○ Exhaustion may affect the body's ability to break down blood clots, according to a study that compared levels of a clot-busting chemical in men who were rested with men who were chronically fatigued. This matters because most heart attacks are caused by a blood clot in the coronary arteries.

○ People with insomnia run a higher risk of developing a major depressive illness over a four-year period than those who sleep well, according to a study by the US National Institute of Mental Health.

○ Men who sleep six hours a night or less, or nine hours or more, are almost twice as likely to die within a nine-year period as men who sleep seven or eight hours a night, according to a study of almost 7000 adults in California.

○ I often doze off when I'm reading, watching television, or in the theater or watching a movie.
○ I avoid activities I like because I feel too tired.

What happens during sleep?

Stacking the zees might seem like a waste of time but it's actually an important physiological and psychological process. It's certainly not simply a 'little death' or a logged-off down-time during which nothing much happens.

Normal sleep can be divided into distinct, highly structured phases:
○ First, you enter a phase called non-rapid eye movement (NREM) sleep (also referred to as slow-wave sleep). Stage 1 of NREM sleep is very light and lasts for just five minutes.
○ Stage 2 NREM sleep is the first part of true sleep and continues for about 10–20 minutes.
○ You then enter Stages 3 and 4 NREM sleep, the deepest part of your sleep; together, these last about 20–40 minutes.
○ This is followed by a return to Stage 2 NREM sleep and then the first phase of rapid eye movement (REM) sleep. This period of REM sleep usually takes place some 70–90 minutes after sleep onset and lasts about 5–15 minutes.
○ NREM and REM cycles alternate throughout the night, although, as sleep progresses, the NREM phases become shorter and the REM phases longer. Overall, 75–80 per cent of total sleep is NREM sleep and 20–25 per cent REM sleep.

It's thought that during periods of NREM sleep, a growth hormone is released into the blood, renewing and restoring body tissues. Athletes experience longer periods of NREM sleep, probably because their bodies need more time to recover from physical stress. During periods of REM sleep, the body is psychologically recuperating, sorting out and storing information as well as working through emotional issues. This is the phase during which most dreaming takes place. REM sleep could be particularly important for memory consolidation: animal experiments show an increase in REM during periods when new behaviors is being learned; if animals are deprived of REM sleep, on the other hand, they learn a new task much less effectively.

I'm dog tired—how can I change?

○ Make more time for sleep. You have to make the decision that it's a priority and simply spend enough time in bed. If you believe that sleep is for wimps, tell yourself that even heavyweight champions make sure they get a good night's sleep before a big fight and that US Army scientists hope to persuade soldiers to nap more in order to maintain their alertness for combat. If you're a bit of an intellectual, on the other hand, model yourself on Albert Einstein—he insisted on 10 hours' sleep a night.

○ Don't forget about napping. Not everyone can manage it, but a daytime nap can make up for lost sleep during the night. But don't sleep for longer than 30 minutes or you'll enter deep sleep and run the risk of feeling groggy when you wake up. (Napping's not a good idea, however, if you have a serious sleep problem: it could make it even harder for you to sleep at night.)

○ Maximize your chances of a restful night's sleep.

Key tips:
  ➲ Avoid caffeine within 4–5 hours of bedtime.
  ➲ Don't eat within two to three hours of going to bed. If you're still digesting food when you lie down you could be kept awake by indigestion or heartburn.
  ➲ Exercise regularly, but not within a couple of hours of bedtime. A US study of over 300 men found that those who took part in regular physical activity enjoyed a significantly lower risk of sleep problems.
  ➲ Avoid alcohol within two hours of bedtime. Although booze can help you fall asleep, it tends to disrupt normal sleep patterns and you're more likely to wake up early when blood alcohol concentrations fall near zero. If you want a night-cap that really will help you sleep, go for a glass of milk. It contains tryptophan, a substance the brain converts into a calm-inducing neurotransmitter called serotonin.
  ➲ Don't get too hot. Your body temperature naturally falls as you approach sleep, and a hot bath or an over-warm bedroom can cause problems. Room temperature should be around 18°C (65°F).
  ➲ Quit smoking. Aside from all its obvious problems, nicotine is a stimulant which can prevent you getting to sleep. Withdrawal symptoms can also wake you up well before the alarm clock.
  ➲ Invest in a comfortable bed and mattress. One study found that, on average, people with uncomfortable beds sleep nearly one hour less than those with comfortable beds.

➲ Avoid reading or watching television in bed. These are waking activities and should be kept separate. You are allowed to have sex in your bedroom, however. In fact, it's recommended as an aid to sleep, whether it's a solo or shared activity.

➲ Avoid late-night arguments with a partner—and if you do have them try to make sure they're resolved before lights-out.

➲ If you're regularly woken up by your children, try establishing shifts with your partner so only one of you loses sleep each night.

○ If you have a sleep problem, take steps to tackle it. If it's long-standing, or is the result of being in pain during the night (perhaps because of backache) or needing to urinate more than once, then see your doctor.

Key tips:

➲ Follow the advice in the previous section.

➲ Wind down during the evening. Impose a deadline of 90 minutes before bedtime for repairs to your house or car, work, and other stimulating activities.

➲ Deal with problems before you go to bed. If you tend to lie awake worrying about the size of your paunch or the state of your bank balance, spend some time earlier in the evening writing down your concerns and a couple of positive steps you can take to sort them out.

➲ Follow a simple relaxation routine both before you go to sleep and if you wake up during the night. Concentrate on breathing in and out slowly and deeply. You could also spend a few minutes tensing and relaxing your major muscle groups: start with your legs; then your stomach and back; arms, neck and shoulders; and, finally, your face and eyes.

➲ Don't try and force yourself to fall asleep. Say to yourself 'Sleep will come when it's ready' or that 'Relaxing in bed is almost as good as sleep'. Keeping your eyes open for a few seconds after they naturally try to close could 'tempt' sleep to take over. If your mind is racing with distracting thoughts, try visualizing a pleasant scene or repeat in your mind a neutral word like 'the'.

➲ If you're not asleep within 20 minutes, get out of bed and sit and relax in another room. Go back to bed only when you feel 'sleepy tired'. This tactic can also help if you wake up for 20 minutes or more during the night.

➲ Meditation can help tackle sleep problems. In one study of people who took an average of 75 minutes to fall asleep, learning to meditate enabled them to drop off after just 15 minutes.

➲ If you're looking for a short-term quick-fix (perhaps because you're going through an unusually stressful time at work), it's worth considering an easily available herbal remedy called valerian. It has a long history of use as a sedative, and, in one study of insomniacs, 89 per cent of users reported improved sleep.

What's stopping you?

I work night shifts and find it hard to get enough sleep
Night-shift workers generally sleep less well than those on day shifts, are more likely to feel tired, and are also prone to a variety of health problems, including peptic ulcers and depression. This is because the body's internal clock finds it extremely difficult to adjust to a new sleep/wake rhythm; in fact, research suggests that shift workers are effectively 'staying up late' rather than actually adapting to night work.

Key tips:
➲ Avoid caffeine during the last half of your shift and fatty food for your last meal before bedtime (it's less digestible). This should make it easier for you to fall asleep when you get home.
➲ Develop a regular sleep pattern. Going to sleep and waking up at different times every day could make your problem even worse.
➲ If you travel home in the morning when it's light, wear dark glasses. (Seriously: bright light has a biological effect, causing the suppression of a sleep-inducing hormone called melatonin.) Make sure your bedroom has thick curtains and, if necessary, wear eye-shades.
➲ If other people are at home when you go to bed, make sure they're as quiet as possible. Bribe them if necessary and/or wear ear-plugs.
➲ If possible, take a short nap in the middle of your shift (but not if you're an airline pilot about to land a jumbo jet).
➲ Don't get trapped in a cycle of drinking loads of caffeine to stay awake at night and drinking alcohol or taking medication to help you sleep during the day. This will ultimately leave you feeling even more strung out.

My partner keeps waking me up because I snore
The two biggest causes of snoring are weight and alcohol. Most serious snorers are overweight and 80 per cent get better if they lose some flab. Alcohol's a problem because it relaxes everything and the tongue can fall back into the neck. Your best bet is to not to drink after 7pm and see if that helps.

BEATING JET LAG

The more time zones you cross, the more your sleep will be affected and the worse you'll feel. But there are ways to help you reset your body clock and hit the ground running.

Key tips:
- ➲ See the light. Bright light can help the body adjust to a new time zone, so make sure you expose yourself to daylight (or other bright light) before your trip.
- ➲ Reschedule your schedule. As soon as you're on the plane, change your watch to your destination time zone. You should then eat and rest as if you were already there.
- ➲ Watch your chow. Overeating, especially rich and fatty foods, will make jet lag feel worse. Refuse the airline stodge and chew your way through a bag of fruit instead.
- ➲ Drink loads. But not booze or coffee. You need stuff that'll keep you well hydrated—a glass of water or orange juice every hour is ideal.
- ➲ Take your trainers. Tests on hamsters show a workout on arrival helps them beat jet lag, and there's anecdotal evidence that the same's true for humans. If you've traveled east, exercise in the morning; if you're traveling west, try it in the late afternoon or early evening.
- ➲ What about drugs? Just say no to sleeping pills—they'll only leave you groggy without helping to reset your body clock. Taking melatonin tablets might help fool your brain into thinking it's bedtime, but they're not available in many countries and there are still doubts about their effectiveness and safety.

If none of this works see your doctor to check whether you could be suffering from a condition known as sleep apnea, in which your breathing regularly stops for 10 seconds or more. One common symptom is that you feel very tired during the day even though you're not aware of any problems at night. Sleep apnea, which affects up to four per cent of men aged 30–50, can sometimes result in high blood pressure, a heart attack, or stroke.

Nightmares keep waking me up

Although we'd probably prefer to dream about long, passionate nights on a desert island with a fantasy lover, up to 10 per cent of us regularly experience nightmares. Typically, they're about feeling helpless in the face of a threat and sometimes involve feeling paralyzed, a sense of falling, being unable to move, or feeling trapped.

Key tips:

➲ Find better ways of dealing with stress while you're awake.

➲ Improve your sleep quality. If you can cut out noise, excessive amounts of alcohol, smoking, and late-night meals, you're less likely to wake up and remember your nightmares.

➲ Check with your doctor about the side-effects of any drugs you're taking.

➲ Tell other people about your nightmares. This could help make them seem less frightening.

➲ Be your own shrink: if you can work out what your nightmares mean, you could try to eliminate the root cause of any anxiety.

➲ Change the nightmare. Before you go to sleep, rehearse the content of your nightmare but change how it ends. For example, instead of staying rooted to the spot, you could fight back and conquer your enemy.

➲ See a professional. If your nightmares are getting you down, or depriving you of too much sleep, it could help to talk to a counselor or psychiatrist.

THINGS YOU DIDN'T KNOW ABOUT SLEEP

○ Simply listening to classical or New Age music before bedtime can help insomnia sufferers, according to a study of a small group of patients in the USA. An overwhelming 96 per cent reported an improvement in their sleep.

○ If you sleep with a partner, you'll almost certainly move around more during the night than if you sleep alone. One study of 46 couples found a strong degree of synchronicity of movement—in other words, when one partner moved, the other soon followed. In mixed-sex couples, there's evidence that it's more common for the man to move first and be followed by his female partner than the other way around. But bed-partners generally sleep better with their companion than on their own.

○ The average adult grows by as much as two centimeters a night. This is simply because the spine is compressed during the day and stretches when it's horizontal. One practical consequence is that you're more likely to injure your back if you exercise with weights soon after you wake up.

○ Sleep is slimming, but unfortunately not for long. Each of us loses up to half a pint of moisture a night (more in hot weather or during illness). But our fluid levels are replenished as soon as we start drinking our breakfast orange juice and coffee.

○ There's no truth is the old adage 'Early to bed and early to rise makes a man healthy, wealthy, and wise.' A long-term UK study of over 1200 men and women found no evidence that people who behave this way earn more, live in better housing, have better mental functioning, or live any longer when compared to people who go to bed and get up later.

CHAPTER 9

PERPETUAL EMOTIONS:
FEELING GOOD ABOUT FEELINGS

There can no longer be any justification for claiming that, when it comes to emotional awareness, men have barely evolved since their ancestors lived in caves and hunted mammoth. In the last 20 years, many more of us have become much more comfortable about expressing our feelings. We're now much less likely to consider it shameful to admit to being scared or vulnerable or even to having a good cry. This greater openness is reflected in men's increasing willingness to use telephone helplines and the steadily growing numbers of men prepared to try counseling. Being able to acknowledge our emotions matters because it can improve our sense of well-being and enable us to build better relationships with others. Recent science also suggests that good emotional health could be as important to good physical health as a nutritious diet and regular exercise.

But many of us can still find emotions hard to handle. We were probably brought up to believe that crying's a 'girl thing' and that boys are supposed to act tough, not soft. It's surely no coincidence that a boy can't buy a miniature therapy couch for his Action Man, only machine guns and bazookas. Even if we do believe it's fine to express feelings, it often feels as if we've got a powerful voice lodged inside our heads constantly reminding us that real men are supposed to maintain a stiff upper lip and a stony silence. We might feel it's okay to express irritability or anger but find it much harder, if not impossible, to show fear or sadness. The good news is that it's not only women's brains that are wired up to handle emotions; just as men are now rapidly learning how to become more active and effective parents, so they can also develop the skills needed to become emotionally healthy.

Why bother with emotions?

○ You'll feel better. The best argument for giving your emotional health a boost is that you'll almost certainly experience more of the pleasant emotions—joy, happiness, contentment, love, and excitement. You'll also be able to deal better with more uncomfortable feelings like shame, guilt and sadness.
○ Your relationships will improve. It's hard to build a good connection with someone who only talks abstractly about work, sport, politics, or his all-consuming interest in collecting fossils. Being able to share how you feel about every aspect of your life, and to empathize with other people's experiences, provides a much better basis for developing solid relationships.
○ You'll achieve more at work. The 21st-century workplace will increasingly depend on emotional skills like good teamwork, excellent communication and the ability to negotiate.
○ You'll cope better with stress. Being able to recognize the signs of stress, and talk about how it feels, are vital ingredients of effective stressbusting.
○ Your mental health will improve. Developing your emotional skills will protect you against common problems like anxiety and depression, and, if you do suffer from them, you're more likely to recover quickly.
○ Your physical health will improve. Simply being open about what you're feeling can boost your immune system, while repressing your feelings weakens it. Men with good mental health are much more likely to be free of heart disease than men who are depressed or anxious.
○ You'll have a better sex life. Living with anxiety and depression can reduce your testosterone levels and sex drive as well as cause problems like erectile dysfunction (impotence).

What is emotional health?

We live in a society where there's more talk than ever of the importance of emotions, where 'ordinary' people reveal their deepest feelings on prime-time television shows like *Oprah* and *Ricki Lake*, and where the sales of self-help books promising instant emotional development are booming. Yet most of us are still brought up to hide our true feelings. We may be scared of how other people will react to our emotional honesty. We might well believe they'll think we're immature, over-emotional, weak, or even crazy. We may also be frightened of other people's emotions, especially if they're strongly expressed, because we're not sure how to respond. Many emotional conflicts, rather than being worked through and resolved,

THE SCIENCE BIT

○ Disclosing emotions boosts the immune system. One study found that when people wrote about their negative experiences for 20 minutes a day for four days, their immune systems functioned better. The greatest improvements occurred among those who wrote about experiences they'd never previously discussed with other people.

○ Suppressing emotional thoughts and expression weakens the immune system, is associated with poorer health, and even an increase in the risk of developing cancer, according to a growing body of research. There's also evidence that trying to repress emotional thoughts is both inherently stressful and ultimately counter-productive because it results in a 'rebound effect'—in other words, the thoughts actually increase in frequency after the period of repression.

○ Emotional disclosure is now known to help with specific illnesses. People with asthma or arthritis who wrote down their feelings about a stressful event in their lives for just 20 minutes on three consecutive days experienced a significant improvement in their condition for up to four months, according to US research. The asthma patients had an average 19 per cent increase in lung function and the arthritis patients had a 28 per cent reduction in the severity of their condition.

○ Expressing anger can reduce the risk of heart disease. A study of 2500 men found that those who let their anger out or who are able to talk about it are up to 75 per cent less likely to develop heart disease than those who repress their anger.

○ Being able to avoid or tackle depression could help you live longer. A large-scale, long-term study suggests that men who don't experience depression are half as likely to develop heart disease or have a heart attack than those who had been seriously depressed at least once. One theory is that depressed people are more likely to develop sticky blood platelets, increasing the risks of blood clots.

end up leading to acts of destruction and violence. Clearly, we don't live in a culture where emotional health is the norm.

There's also a widely-held view that good emotional health is about being happy all the time. There's certainly nothing wrong with happiness—it is, of course, a highly desirable emotion—but it's completely unrealistic to believe that anyone can exist in a

REAL HEALTH FOR MEN

state of permanent nirvana. Sometimes it's actually extremely important for us to feel unhappy: after a bereavement or relationship breakdown, for example, feelings of sadness, anger, and depression are natural and essential elements of the process of coming to terms with the loss of a loved one. Similarly, before an examination or a job interview, feelings of anxiety or fear are not only normal but they can also help to improve our performance. Some psychologists believe that striving to achieve a state of constant joy or happiness can result in the denial or repression of very important feelings like guilt, anger, sadness, or grief. One consequence is that we ultimately feel even worse, not only because it's impossible to ignore uncomfortable feelings forever but because we can also end up feeling a failure for having them in the first place.

The key to better emotional health is not to try to limit the range of feelings we experience, but rather to develop the skills we need to deal effectively with the feelings we have about our relationships, work, family, and every other aspect of life. To achieve this, we need to:

○ Recognize, understand, and express the full range of our feelings.
○ Know how to manage our emotions appropriately (so we don't start shouting at, or even hitting, everyone who disagrees with us).
○ Be able to empathize with other people and to interact with them emotionally.
○ Acquiring this package of skills, sometimes referred to as 'emotional literacy' or 'emotional intelligence', will provide us with the resources to cope well with the bad times and to enjoy the good.

My emotions are more blocked than my nose —how can I change?

○ Decide you want to. If you think you're currently emotionally numb, or that your emotional range is too limited, ask yourself whether you'd prefer to stay that way or to discover the full range of human passions. The risk of changing is that you could start to experience emotions that are sometimes confusing, unpleasant, or even overwhelming. On the other hand, you may sense that continuing as you are means you're missing out on valuable and enriching experiences. But becoming emotionally literate is a process requiring both courage and commitment. Emotional repression is as difficult a habit to break as smoking—perhaps even harder because you've probably been doing it for much longer. And unlike quitting cigarettes, becoming more emotionally literate cannot be achieved by will-power alone. It's a skill, and, like most skills (whether it's windsurfing, playing the guitar, or ten-pin bowling), it can only be done well if it's practiced, practiced, and practiced.

EMOTIONS—WHO NEEDS THEM?

You might sometimes feel as if life would be a lot easier if we were all Vulcans like Mr. Spock in *Star Trek* and could successfully repress all our emotions or simply not have them in the first place. But, aside from the fact that it's impossible to abolish feelings, they are extremely important to our well-being. Becoming purely rational, non-emotional beings wouldn't actually help us much; we ignore our feelings at our peril—literally.

In his book *Emotional Intelligence*, Daniel Goleman suggests there are at least four core emotions: fear, anger, sadness, and enjoyment. At or near the core are several other key emotions, including love, surprise, disgust, and shame. Each of these emotions is surrounded by three other emotional states: 'moods,' which are more muted and last for longer than a core emotion; 'temperaments,' a near-constant state of readiness for a particular emotion or mood; and 'disorders,' a condition in which someone becomes trapped in an emotional state.

Core emotion	Mood	Temperament	Disorder
Fear	Anxious,	Nervous, wary, apprehensive	Phobic, panicked edgy
Anger	Annoyed	Irritable, grumpy hateful or violent	Pathologically
Sadness	Sorrowful, despairing	Lonely, dejected, gloomy	Depressed
Enjoyment	Happy, joyful	Contented	Manic

Some psychologists argue that these emotions haven't evolved by accident. Fear, for example, exists to alert us to risk and danger; when we first feel it, we tend to freeze—perhaps to give us time to decide whether we should run away, hide, or fight—and then blood rushes to the large skeletal muscles enabling us to implement whatever decision we've made. Anger, too, generates a rush of hormones, increased blood flow, and a surge of energy, increasing our ability to fight. Sadness slows the body's metabolism and depletes energy levels, enabling us to remain near home and in safety while we adjust to a bereavement or major disappointment. Enjoyment, on the other hand, produces increased activity in an area of the brain that inhibits negative feelings and creates a readiness and enthusiasm for the task at hand.

EMOTIONS—WHO NEEDS THEM?

The role of the other central emotions is also clear. Disgust—a response to an unpleasant taste or smell—warns us to avoid or reject contaminated food. Surprise lifts the eyebrows and widens the eyes, enabling us to process more information about an unexpected event and assess the best possible response. Love also has its uses: tender feelings and sexual satisfaction create restorative feelings of calm and contentment and facilitate co-operation between people.

Trying to operate without emotions would be as hard as attempting to function without intelligence. In fact, our emotions and our intellect have to work together to enable us to understand what's going on in the environment and decide how to react.

○ Remember that there's no right or wrong way to have feelings. Because men are often criticized by women for not expressing their feelings, it can sometimes seem as if we should be expressing our feelings in exactly the same way as them. Not so. First, there's actually no such thing as a 'female way' of expressing feelings: it's pretty obvious that individual women vary enormously in the way they handle their emotions. Secondly, and more importantly, each man will almost certainly benefit most from finding a way of dealing with his emotions that feels right and comfortable for him.

○ Focus on your feelings. If you find it hard to get in touch with your emotions, you might find the following exercise a helpful first step.

➲ Stop whatever you're doing. Lie down somewhere comfortable. Take several deep, slow breaths, close your eyes, and relax. Don't worry—you're not about to be asked to embark on some wacky mystical experience.

➲ Now think back over the last 24 hours. Pick out several events—they don't have to be anything particularly unusual or remarkable—and try to remember them in as much detail as you can.

➲ As you run over what happened, try to recall how you felt at the time. When you were nearly getting knocked off your bicycle by a careless driver, perhaps you felt a mixture of fear and anger. When your boss dismissed your ideas during a key meeting at work, maybe you felt useless and worthless. When you walked down a crowded street and noticed that all your trouser buttons were undone, you might have felt seriously embarrassed. As you remember these events, you may well have some further feelings about them; try to focus on these too and become aware of what they are. If you find it hard to describe how you're feeling, the following list might help.

50 EMOTIONS

aggressive	decisive	flat	lonely	satisfied
angry	depressed	frightened	negative	sexy
anxious	desirable	fulfilled	numb	shy
aroused	despairing	guilty	positive	tense
ashamed	disgusted	happy	powerful	ugly
attractive	disturbed	hollow	powerless	upset
bored	elated	important	reckless	useless
brave	embarrassed	indecisive	relaxed	virile
calm	excited	in love	restless	withdrawn
confident	exhausted	irritable	sad	worthless

➲ Repeat this exercise several times until you can begin to identify at least some of your feelings. You can then take the opportunity to try regular 'refresher' exercises at almost any time, perhaps while you're sitting on a train on your way to work.

➲ Also, try paying attention to how you're feeling when you're engaged in an activity that can generate strong emotions, perhaps reading a novel, listening to music, watching a film, waiting to see the dentist, or even taking a ride on the gravity-defying and heart-stopping big dipper at your local funfair.

○ Learn the difference between thoughts and feelings. Men are often brilliant at abstract thought, but because they can find it harder to be aware of what they're feeling, they sometimes get the two mixed up. A thought is a judgement, interpretation, or opinion of an event, whereas a feeling is your emotional response.

➲ Thoughts include statements like 'I think you're an idiot' or 'I feel that you're an idiot'. Even though the second statement includes the word 'feel,' what's being said actually reflects an interpretation or judgement. Statements like 'I feel you should see your mother more often' or 'When you spoke to me after our argument I felt you were angry' are also thoughts, not feelings.

➲ Feelings include statements like 'I feel angry', 'I feel worried,' or 'I feel happy.' Strictly speaking, when people say they feel 'humiliated,' 'rejected,' 'insulted,' or 'loved,' they are describing thoughts, not feelings. That's because these are their interpretations of what they believe others are doing to them. The true feeling is usually hidden beneath the thought—for instance, it might be more accurate to say 'I think you are rejecting me and that makes me feel sad and lonely.'

➲ Feelings often also have a physical component; thoughts don't. If you feel embarrassed, for instance, your cheeks will often feel warm; if you feel frightened, your knees might well go wobbly; if you feel angry, your muscles could tense up.

○ As you develop a clearer understanding of what constitutes a genuine feeling, it should become easier to become more aware of your emotional state.

➲ Write your feelings down. Start a journal in which you keep a regular record of how you feel about the different aspects of your life, including your work, your friendships, your relationships, and your interests and hobbies. If you feel sad when your football team loses, write it down; if you feel elated when you get a pay rise at work, make sure all the details are included. Because nobody need see your journal, you can be as honest as you feel able.

➲ Say 'I feel'. When you're talking (or writing) about your feelings, actually say 'I feel that ...' rather than 'I think that ...' or 'I believe that ...' The more you use the language of feelings, the easier it can become to feel them.

➲ Start small. If you're not used to sharing your feelings, it might be best not to start by telling your family precisely why they irritate you so much. You might be better off beginning with telling your partner or a friend how you feel about a movie, a book, or a piece of music. If you do want to tell other people how you feel about them, try starting with what you like about them. It needn't be a big thing, perhaps their taste in clothes or that they make excellent coffee.

➲ Be honest. It's actually better to say nothing than to be emotionally phoney. Fake feelings will confuse whoever you're talking to and make it harder for you to be clear about what you really feel.

⮑ Learn to listen to other people's feelings. Even though it's easy to switch off when you hear things that make you feel uncomfortable, awkward, embarrassed, or simply bored, you can learn a great deal from discovering how other people experience their feelings. What's more, it's difficult to empathize with other people—a crucial tool in your emotional repertoire—if you don't even listen to what's being said. When other people share their feelings with you, show that you've heard and understood what they've disclosed. It's often better to say something like 'Yes, I can appreciate how you feel' than to start offering practical advice in an attempt to provide a quick fix.

⮑ Experiment with people you know and trust. There's little point in practicing talking about your feelings to people who might put you down and reinforce the idea that you're a sissy for even mentioning an emotion. This could mean keeping your mouth shut when you're having a beer with your mates after your weekly soccer match but deciding to be more expressive when you're on your own with a more responsive friend.

⮑ Notice your emotional controls. These are techniques most of us use, almost always without being aware of it, to repress our emotions. The main controls include:

    ○ Denial. We pretend to ourselves and others that we're not feeling anything and hope that the feeling will soon go away.

    ○ Avoidance. We switch our attention to something else every time we feel an emotion we're not comfortable with.

    ○ Numbing out. We use drugs, alcohol, food, or sex to blot out our feelings.

The more open and honest you can become, the easier it will be to spot when you're trying to control your emotions in any of these ways. You can then try to remain open to your feelings instead.

○ Manage your feelings. While it's important to be open and honest, it's also vital to take responsibility for your feelings. Just because you're trying to express yourself doesn't give you the right to hurt other people, either emotionally or physically.

Key tips:

⮑ Avoid judging or accusing other people when you feel bad. When you're upset, it's easy to say things like 'You behaved like a bastard by so rudely ignoring me at work yesterday,' but these sorts of blaming statements almost always cause the other person to reply in kind, leading to a vicious circle of accusation and counter-accusation. It might be better to say something like 'When you didn't speak to me at work yesterday, I felt upset and then angry'. This response contains a fact—you weren't spoken to—and a statement of your feelings. It also avoids any speculative interpretation of the other person's motives and makes it easier for him or her to respond in a way that leads to dialogue rather than confrontation.

➲ It's fine to get angry, but don't get aggressive. It's easy to believe that anger can only be expressed by shouting, screaming, and even physical violence. This isn't true. Anger can be expressed in many other, much more productive ways. Simply telling people you're angry is important—you don't have to whisper it but you don't have to bang your fist on the table either. If you feel as if you are about to be violent, you can always decide to walk away immediately and not return until you've calmed down.

➲ Choose your moment. It's possible to feel something strongly but not express it immediately. In fact, most of us do this all the time: if we're feeling angry with our boss, for example, we're not likely to show it if there's a good chance we'll end up without a job. It can make much more sense to reveal how we're feeling at a time when the other person is able to listen and respond.

○ Boost your self-esteem. Being honest and open about feelings can seem a risky business; it can make anyone feel distinctly vulnerable, especially at first. If you feel stupid or worthless, you may well assume that nobody will be interested in what you have to say. It can be much easier, therefore, if you have some sense of your own value and significance. Having a higher level of self-esteem can also help you recover faster from emotional setbacks. For instance, if your partner has just left you, you may well feel rejected and lonely. That's perfectly normal and natural. But if you feel basically good about yourself, you'll also appreciate that you have the capacity to form another relationship and probably won't spend the rest of your life on your own.

Key tips:
➲ Think about the origins of any negative feelings you have about yourself. You weren't born with low self-esteem; in fact, as a baby, you were biologically programmed to act as if you were the most important being in the universe. We acquire low self-esteem as a result of our experiences with parents, teachers, and our peers as well as the wider world. Some religious authorities may even have told us that we were born bad or sinful. Identifying the causes of low self-esteem can help us understand that it's not an inherent part of our psychological make-up.

➲ If you suffer from low self-esteem, compare what you feel about yourself with evidence that suggests the opposite. You may feel stupid, for example, but is there any evidence that this might not in fact be the case? What about some good examination results, your expertise at your hobbies, or the positive things people sometimes say about you? If you feel worthless, is there any evidence that you have made some sort of positive contribution to the lives of people you know or the work you do? Even if you have experienced some serious setbacks in your life, the chances are that the negative image you have of yourself is still a distorted one.

➲ Take yourself more seriously. Try treating yourself as you would like other people to treat you. This could mean not putting yourself down, behaving more like an adult than a child, and trusting your own judgement. Taking better care of your health is one important way in which you can feel better about yourself. It may also help if you can take steps to improve your body image (see Chapter 15). If you spend time with people who have got into the habit of mocking you—or worse—then let them know how it makes you feel or try to develop a new, and more respectful, circle of friends.

➲ Be more rounded. This doesn't mean putting on weight. Rather, psychologists have discovered that someone's sense of identity and self-esteem is more likely to be fragile if it's based on just one or two areas of life. This could be a particular problem for men who have become very focused on work: if they lose their job, their self-esteem plummets. Your self-esteem could become much more robust if it's rooted in many aspects of your life—perhaps an intimate relationship, family, friends, sports, and cultural interests as well as work.

➲ Be more assertive. This has nothing to do with aggression. It's about being explicit about your needs, stating them clearly, and then negotiating an acceptable compromise. Let's say your boss wants you to spend two days traveling abroad to a crucial meeting with a new client. But your partner's recovering from a serious illness and you want to be able to go home every evening to cook, clean, and be an all-round Florence Nightingale. Non-assertive responses could include agreeing to your boss's request, even though you know you'd feel worried and guilty while you were away. Alternatively, you might become angry or intimidating in an attempt to get her to change her mind. The assertive response would be to explain the position to your boss, make it clear you'd be happy to go a few weeks later, or suggest other possible solutions to the problem (e.g. you could identify other members of staff who might make the trip, arrange a tele-conference link-up with the client, or suggest your firm pays for the client to visit you). Even if your boss is initially frustrated or disappointed by your inability to travel, there's a good chance that a mutually acceptable compromise can be achieved.

➲ Accept you'll feel bad about yourself at times. No matter how robust your self-esteem, there's a good chance that you'll occasionally feel stupid, ugly, or incompetent. What's important is to understand that these feelings don't represent fundamental truths about yourself. But it's also important to understand that your feelings may be telling you that something does need to change. If you're sacked for being bad at your job, for instance, you may have to accept that your employer's behavior was justified. Being sacked doesn't mean that you're a failure to the core of your being but it may mean that you need to learn some new skills if you want to get—and hold onto—another job.

➲ Don't put other people down in an attempt to make yourself feel better. It's a tempting strategy and many people try it, but it's usually counter-productive. You'll probably only end up feeling guilty, ashamed, and generally even worse about yourself.

○ Consider seeing a counselor or therapist. You might think that seeing an 'emotions expert' is necessary only if you have some sort of serious psychological problem. While it's true that most people seek counseling because they're experiencing some sort of emotional crisis, it's perfectly possible and acceptable to see a counselor to explore your past, work out how it's affecting you now, and to find ways of improving the quality of your life. This process could help you understand much more about your feelings and enable you to express them much more easily and fully.

Tackling depression

Depression is a very common problem among men—one study found that one in 12 suffers from major depression—and the number affected is probably increasing steadily. One key factor could be recent changes in the roles of men and women: the fall in the number of men in full-time work, and the increase in the numbers of working women, have resulted in many men experiencing a loss of status and becoming socially isolated.

It's recently been recognized that men can get the baby blues, too. While post-natal depression is much more common in women, a study of 200 couples found that up to nine per cent of fathers can be affected six weeks after the birth and five per cent six months after the birth. A man is particularly susceptible if his partner is experiencing depression, but it's also likely that a major risk factor for the modern

FINDING A COUNSELOR OR THERAPIST

Given the explosion in interest in emotional self-exploration over the last 20 years, it's now easier than ever to find a good counselor.

Key tips:
- ➤ Contact professional counseling organizations which can send you a list of qualified counsellors in your area. They can also give you information about the different approaches to counseling to enable you to decide which appeals to you most.
- ➤ Decide whether you'd prefer to see a man or woman or whether this doesn't matter.
- ➤ Think about whether you'd prefer to work one-to-one with a counselor or in a larger group. Group counseling has the advantage of being cheaper and can help you understand more about how you behave with other people, as well as giving you useful insights into other people's psyches.
- ➤ Phone up counsellors and explain what you're after and ask them about their approach. Make sure you understand the level of commitment they'll expect you to make and how much they charge.
- ➤ Arrange an initial, one-off counseling session. Although you'll probably have to pay for this, you're under no obligation to go back if it doesn't feel right.

The terms 'counseling' and 'therapy' tend to be used interchangeably, although sometimes counseling is used to mean shorter-term and therapy longer-term work.

father is the contradictory pressures he experiences to be both a provider for his family and an actively involved parent.

The key symptoms of depression are:
- ○ Feeling unhappy, miserable, depressed, or numb.
- ○ The inability to enjoy anything.
- ○ Being unable to concentrate properly.
- ○ Feeling guilty about things that have nothing to do with you.
- ○ Experiencing difficulties in getting to sleep.
- ○ Waking early or during the night.
- ○ A loss of interest in sex.
- ○ Losing weight.

○ Performing less well at work.
○ Becoming unusually withdrawn, quiet, and feeling unable to talk.
○ Worrying more than usual.
○ Feeling more irritable than usual.
○ Complaining more about vague physical symptoms.

Almost everybody will experience some of these symptoms for a while, usually for a good reason (e.g. because of a bereavement or a relationship breakdown). They become a serious problem if they continue for a long time and take over your life.

Key tips:
➲ Remember that being depressed doesn't mean you're weak. Depression is no better or worse than catching flu or breaking your arm; it certainly isn't a reflection on your masculinity. It might help you to know that Winston Churchill suffered regular bouts of intense depression but was still able to be an effective leader of his country, even during wartime.
➲ Try to talk about how you feel. It's extremely easy to become completely closed in by your problems. If someone takes the time to listen to you and to acknowledge your difficulties, it validates you as a person and can help put your feelings into perspective.
➲ Chill out. Relaxation techniques can help reduce feelings of tension (see Chapter 10).
➲ Exercise. It's been shown to be at least as effective as psychotherapy in tackling moderate depression.
➲ Avoid alcohol or drugs. They may make you feel better for a few hours but will probably make you feel worse in the long run. Any addictive behaviors, including gambling, sex, or using pornography, is likely to have the same effect.
➲ Give it some herbal. Even hardened critics of complementary medicine are hard-pressed to deny the effectiveness of a plant known as St John's wort (*Hypericum perforatum*) in tackling mild or moderately severe depression. A review of 23 clinical trials involving over 1750 people found the herb to be significantly superior to a placebo (a dummy drug) and as effective as standard anti-depressants. What's more, it has few side-effects and won't affect your driving.
➲ See your doctor. He or she may be able to refer you to a counselor or prescribe anti-depressant drugs. These can be remarkably effective, although they can have side-effects. Prozac, for example, frequently causes mild sickness, diarrhea, headaches, and insomnia.

Are you having a mid-life crisis?

It's becoming clear that many men experience a range of emotional problems for a period between the ages of about 35 and 60. This has become known as the 'mid-life crisis'. The main symptoms include:

○ Increased irritability.
○ Indecisiveness.
○ Anxiety.
○ Depression.
○ Loss of self-confidence.
○ Loss of a sense of direction in life.
○ Feeling lonely and unattractive.
○ Forgetfulness.
○ Difficulty concentrating.
○ Fears about sexual decline.
○ An increase in sexual fantasies.
○ Increased relationship problems.

Some doctors believe the mid-life crisis is chiefly a physiological problem—due mainly to a decline in 'bio-available' testosterone (see page 259)—but most argue that the causes are primarily psychological. These include:

○ Realizing you're no longer young and that your youth has gone forever. Your body in particular is increasingly showing the signs of ageing.
○ Discovering you're not immortal. The death or serious illness of a parent or a male friend can make you feel as if you could be next. You may even have started to experience some worrying health problems of your own.
○ Relationship problems. As you contemplate what it will be like growing old with your partner, you may become increasingly aware of any difficulties you have with the relationship. These can become more exposed if you have children who have recently left home.
○ Work problems. As the workplace changes rapidly and new skills are in demand, you may feel as if it's increasingly difficult for you to maintain your position and income. You may believe your most successful years are now behind you.

The journey from youth to middle-age and on into old age may seem frightening and painful, but you can also see it as an opportunity to re-evaluate and perhaps change the direction of your life. Rather than believing that ageing is simply about having to give things up, try to think about what you'd like to start. When you reach 60, you could still be only two-thirds of the way through your life. That leaves a great deal of time to broaden your interests, travel, return to education, learn new work skills or take up new sports. Don't forget that Everest was climbed by a 60-year-old in 1999.

But it's also important not to pretend that you feel simply great about ageing. You may need to spend time accepting that many of your aspirations may now remain unrealized. You may never have a body like Brad Pitt's, you may never become chief of a multinational corporation, and you may never have sex with 10 lovers simultaneously. It's important to try to talk about how you feel, whether it's to a partner, friend, or counselor.

What's stopping you?

Only sissies talk about their feelings

It's certainly true that the fear of being called a sissy has led many men to bottle up their emotions. Men are, at least traditionally, supposed to be tough, stoical, and rational; they are not supposed to reveal their fear, vulnerability, or weakness. This may have been useful in an era when men's primary role was to hunt and fight, but it is surely redundant in the 21st century. Not only does emotional repression affect men's health, it also limits their relationships with other men and women and affects their ability to perform effectively at work. There are so many good arguments for men learning to broaden their emotional repertoire that it's now a bigger sign of weakness to decide not to do so.

I just feel numb

You're not alone—in fact, doctors have a term, alexithymia, to describe a state of emotional numbness. One psychologist has estimated that as many as 80 per cent of men have a mild to severe form of it. Feeling numb is often a symptom of depression, and, since sharing feelings is one of the best treatments for depression, you could try talking about your sense of emotional numbness. What's it really like? How long have you felt this way? Do you remember a time when you didn't feel numb? Do you have any idea why you might have started to feel numb? If talking doesn't work, you could try a self-help medication like St John's wort or see a doctor for something stronger.

QUICK WAYS TO MAKE YOURSELF FEEL BETTER

Are you feeling a bit jaded, a touch blue, or a little out of sorts? Are you fed up with being irritable, concerned that life's lost its sparkle, or worried since your friends started calling you Mr. Grumpy? Here are some cheap, easy and effective ways to bring back Mr.Happy. (Guaranteed side-effect free.)

CHANGE YOUR GRUB

When you're feeling low, your thoughts may well turn to cakes and chocolate. But you're much more likely to get a mental boost from foods high in carbohydrate rather than fat—and that means plenty of healthy potatoes, pasta, rice, and cereals. Fat can make you feel tired and dreamy, but carbohydrate boosts blood-sugar levels and energy levels. A high carbohydrate meal also stimulates the brain's production of serotonin, a key neurotransmitter which plays an important role in mood. If you want to feel attentive, vigorous, and assertive, there are few better ways of starting the day than tucking into a high-carbohydrate, low-fat breakfast—that means cereal, bread, and fruit.

GET OFF YER BUTT

If the word 'exercise' reminds you of running round cold school gyms or humiliation in communal showers, you might be surprised to learn that a bit of physical activity is good for the mind as well as the body. In a study of healthy volunteers working out on a HealthRider (a cross between an exercise bike and a rowing machine), sports scientists at Birmingham University in the UK noticed significant psychological benefits from moderate exercise for 30 minutes three times a week. As the tests progressed, the volunteers' confidence grew, not just in their capacity for exercise but in their ability to tackle everyday situations. They were less irritable, believed their energy levels to be higher, and generally felt better about themselves.

HAVE SEX

If you've got a sexual problem—perhaps impotence, premature ejaculation, or a low sex drive—then you should head for a doctor or sex therapist before trying a work-out between the sheets. But if your organs are up to speed, it's worth knowing that sex creates similar physiological changes to exercise. You'll use the same amount of energy during an hour's passionate sex (if you're lucky enough to last that long) as you would in the first half of a soccer match, so a good

QUICK WAYS TO MAKE YOURSELF FEEL BETTER

session in the sack could release just as many mood-enhancing brain chemicals. Sex can also produce a sense of intimacy and self-affirmation that results in a significant boost to self-esteem.

WRITE A POEM

Your partner's walked out, someone's smashed into your car, and your boss has told you to clear your desk by the end of the week. Not surprisingly, you're feeling a bit low. Try writing a poem about it. No kidding. Over half of those taking part in a study at Bristol University in the UK found it was a useful outlet for their emotions and helped them cope better with stress. Almost as many said reading poetry also helped, so dust off those Wordsworth sonnets.

HAVE A LAUGH

Mirthful laughter is known to lower stress-hormone levels and boost your immunity. Acting like a mini-workout, a good session of side-splitting humor also speeds up the heart rate and circulation as well as boosting oxygen intake and reducing muscle tension. Laughter also releases endorphins, the body's natural pain killers. It's been estimated that, on average, men laughed for 18 minutes a day in the 1950s and for only six minutes a day in the 1990s, so it's probably time to switch off those gloomy television documentaries and head for the local video shop's comedy section.

THINK ABOUT IT

Meditation definitely isn't just for Tibetan monks. There's increasingly compelling evidence of its effectiveness in improving mental and physical health. One of the most studied forms, transcendental meditation (TM), can provide an impressive range of benefits and life-enhancing effects. Regularly practiced, TM has been shown to reduce anxiety and mild depression, improve insomnia and tension headaches, and help with a range of stress-related conditions.

TRY A MASSAGE

Get a massage, from a professional practitioner, a partner, or your own hands. Research shows it can significantly reduce stress and anxiety in cancer patients and it's now increasingly being used within orthodox medicine. Massaging the ears can help tackle tiredness and has a generally stimulating effect on the body

QUICK WAYS TO MAKE YOURSELF FEEL BETTER

and mind; pressing the acupuncture point in the groove just below the nose improves concentration; and deeply massaging the center of your palm helps relieve anxiety. Using essential oils—particularly clary sage or ylang ylang—with massage could also make a difference.

FACE THOSE DEMONS

When you feel low, it's easy to try to ignore what's happening or simply accept it as inevitable. But there's a better mental strategy. An investigation by psychologists at Leicester University in the UK into the techniques people use to improve their mood found the two most frequently mentioned were 'confrontation' (e.g. making plans to solve the problem) and 'positive distraction' (e.g. fantasizing about pleasant things). When, in a follow-up study, people were asked to use just one of these strategies whenever they experienced an unpleasant mood or emotion, confrontation proved the most effective. And this doesn't have to be done in isolation: talking to someone who listens, empathizes, and perhaps even suggests practical solutions can help enormously.

THINGS YOU DIDN'T KNOW ABOUT EMOTIONS

○ Women cry five times more often than men, according to a study of 448 British and Israeli men and women aged 20–42. Just four per cent of the men said they cried frequently or very frequently compared to 22 per cent of the women; 62 per cent of the men said they never or almost never cried, compared to 11 per cent of the women.

○ Some scientists believe that one reason why people tend to feel better after crying is that stress chemicals are actually removed from the body in tears. One study even found that those suffering from stress-related illnesses like ulcers and colitis were much less likely to cry than healthy people of the same sex and age. Three quarters of men say they feel better after crying.

○ If you believe in the 'Monday Blues' you're much more likely to experience them. Psychologists have found that if people are told they're more likely to feel in a bad mood on Mondays then they will feel worse than people who've been told that the Monday Blues are a myth.

CHAPTER 10

RELAX, MAN:
TURNING DISTRESS INTO DE-STRESS

en are feeling more and more stressed. We're now expected to work long hours in increasingly demanding and insecure jobs, devote more time to our relationships, and be involved and active fathers. And we're supposed to find enough spare time to exercise until we have the body of an Adonis. It's not surprising that 49 per cent of us say we generally feel stressed out, according to a survey by a UK men's health magazine. Work is the biggest cause of men's stress, followed by home relationships and money; 42 per cent claim that their sexual performance has been affected, while 32 per cent have turned to alcohol as a way of coping. This matters because stress not only feels, er, stressful, it's also a serious health risk.

While many men are beginning to recognize that stress is causing them problems, others are still reluctant to admit it. Perhaps this isn't so surprising since most of us have been brought up to believe that only wimps get stressed. Let's face it, you'd be very surprised if Captain Kirk left the bridge of the Starship *Enterprise* before commencing battle with the Klingons because he'd developed a bout of stress-related diarrhea. As we know from countless war films and westerns, real men don't get stressed, they just get going. Most of us aren't like that, of course, however much we might want to be. Rather than pretending that we can effortlessly tackle whatever life throws at us, we might be better off accepting the reality of stress and looking for methods of coping better. Fortunately, there are many effective ways to beat stress—and none of them involves spending hours lying on a bed of nails or swimming with dolphins (however delightful that might be).

THE SCIENCE BIT

○ Stress increases the risk of catching a cold. In a US study, healthy volunteers were exposed to a virus that causes the common cold. Although 84 per cent of the participants were infected by the virus, only 40 per cent developed colds. Those who reported being exposed to chronic life stressors (ones lasting at least one month) were more likely to succumb to the cold virus than those who said they'd been exposed to only acute stressful events (lasting less than one month).

○ The better you can cope with stress, the less likely you are to develop an ulcer in the stomach or duodenum. A US study of over 4500 adults previously free of ulcers found that those who described themselves as stress-free were about half as likely to develop an ulcer as those who described themselves as stressed. Those who felt unstressed were three times less likely to develop an ulcer than the most stressed.

○ Stress is a factor in depression. Forty-two per cent of men believe stress at work triggered a period of depression, according to a survey by the Depression Alliance in the UK. A study which compared depressed American patients with similar non-depressed people found that the depressed group had recently experienced significantly more stressful life events.

○ Stress is linked to cancer. In a US study, 110 men with suspected but unconfirmed lung cancer were psychologically assessed. Each was later diagnosed as having either cancer or a benign tumor. The men who'd recently suffered psychological stresses such as job instability or relationship breakdown were more likely to have cancer. Psychological factors were as accurate as a history of smoking at predicting who would develop cancer.

○ Stress is bad for the heart. If patients with coronary artery disease are given stressful tasks like mental arithmetic or speaking publicly on a personal subject, over half of them will suffer a rise in blood pressure and abnormal movements in the heart wall. Other research found that asking cardiac patients to remember a recent event that made them angry induces constrictions in their coronary arteries.

○ Stress might even kill you. A Swedish study of 750 middle-aged men found that those experiencing stressful life events in the previous year were much more likely to die from any cause in the following seven years. Experiencing divorce or separation increased the risk of death more than three times, feeling insecure at work increased it by two-and-a-half times. Those men who'd experienced three or more stressful life events were almost four times as likely to die than those who'd remained stress free.

Why bother to tackle stress?

○ You'll feel better. If you can manage your stress more effectively, you'll sleep more soundly, have more energy, and suffer from fewer headaches, nervous twitches, or stomach upsets.

○ Your relationships could improve. As your stress levels fall, you'll be less irritable and angry and altogether a much nicer person to talk to and spend time with.

○ Your sex life will get a boost. Stress certainly isn't an aphrodisiac. It depletes your sex hormones and is a major cause of sexual problems such as erectile dysfunction (impotence), loss of desire, and premature ejaculation.

○ You'll take better care of your health. It's easier to tackle problems like drinking too much alcohol, smoking, or overeating if your stress levels are under control.

○ You'll be healthier. If you reduce your susceptibility to stress, you'll also cut your risk of developing a wide range of diseases ranging from the common cold to cancer. You'll probably also live longer.

What is stress?

You know what it's like. It's already 4pm and you've got to finish a report for your boss by the end of the day. You missed lunch so you feel drained and hungry, the computer's just crashed for the third time, and your phone won't stop ringing. Your head already feels as if it's about to explode when your partner calls to remind you not to forget the shopping for tonight's dinner. As you realize you can't get everything done, you even begin to feel stressed about feeling stressed. It doesn't take much longer before you finally reach breaking point—as your colleagues discover when they hear you giving your filing cabinet a good kicking. Not every experience of stress is this dramatic, of course, but even minor symptoms can quickly escalate.

Stress isn't so much about what happens to us but how we *feel* about what happens to us. To take one example, politicians are normally quite relaxed about appearing on television to justify their policies, however absurd those policies might be. Most of the rest of us, however, would probably get so panicked by the thought of having to defend ourselves before an audience of millions that we'd feel like swallowing a bucketful of tranquilizers or hiding in a cupboard until the program's over. We all react differently to what psychologists call 'life events,' and, clearly, events that are stressful for one person may not be stressful for another.

This suggests that there's nothing inevitable about feeling stressed. If politicians can feel good about appearing on television then this demonstrates that it's not in

STRESS-RELATED SYMPTOMS

Emotional	Muscular	Organs	Behavior
Anxiety	Trembling hands	Flushing/flashing	Insomnia
Worry	Fidgeting	Sweating	Clumsiness
Over-excitement	Nervous twitches	Light-headedness	Higher levels of smoking, drinking, taking drugs, etc.
Forgetfulness	Tense muscles	Dry mouth	Making mistakes
Confusion	Grinding teeth	Cold hands and feet	Becoming withdrawn
Concentration problems	Clenched jaw	Frequent urination	Increased (or decreased) appetite
Irritability	Headaches	Diarrhea	Sexual problems
Boredom	Pounding heart	Constipation	Short-temper
Apathy	Rapid breathing	Upset stomach	Sleeping more (or less)

Note: All these symptoms can also be caused by non-stress-related problems.
If they persist, be sure to get medical advice.

fact an inherently stressful experience. Indeed, it might even be possible for any of us to feel as comfortable in a television studio as we do in our living room at home.

Most of us have probably already experienced how our feelings can change about an event that once seemed stressful. A man about to make his first parachute jump is likely to feel stressed to the point of near terror, for example, even if he's very good at hiding it. He'll be breathing rapidly, his heart will be pounding, the palms of his hands will be sweating and he'll probably have made a hundred trips to the toilet. But by his third or fourth jump, he'll probably feel a lot more relaxed—he'll be waving to his mates on the way down, taking photographs, and generally having a good time.

In fact, the politician on television and the experienced skydiver almost certainly experience some stress, but it's the kind that gives them a buzz and feels positive. The extra alertness and energy it provides may even help to improve their performance. A certain level of stress is, in fact, necessary for all of us to function effectively, and without it we'd probably soon feel completely unchallenged and unstimulated. The key is control. If we feel we can cope with the events we're experiencing then they're tolerable, sometimes even exciting. But when the pressure builds up to a point where we begin to feel things are spinning out of control, then we start to experience those all-too familiar—and very unpleasant—stress symptoms.

The biology of stress

Our bodies react to any life-threatening or hazardous challenge by channeling their resources to deal with the threat.

- Because the obvious solution is usually to fight or flee, the adrenal glands (which are located next to the kidneys) immediately release the hormone adrenaline. This increases the speed and force of the heartbeat, widens the airways to increase the intake of oxygen and narrows blood vessels in the skin and intestines so that an increased flow of blood reaches the brain and muscles.
- The adrenal glands then release extra amounts of the hormone cortisol to help convert the body's energy reserves of fat and carbohydrate into a form suitable for immediate use by the brain and muscles.
- Endorphins are released from the brain and elsewhere which act like opiate drugs in reducing the perception of pain. That's why people who suffer severe injuries often can't feel them.
- The stress response boosts the body's immune system, at least in the short term. That's useful if you're injured running from or fighting with a predator (whether it's a lion in Africa or the wasps' nest you ill-advisedly tried to remove from your loft).
- In the longer-term, however, the stress response starts to deplete the immune system; cortisol and the endorphins have a particularly damaging effect. This means the body is more susceptible to invading microbes and less able to detect and destroy developing tumors.
- As part of the body's mobilization of its fuel reserves, fatty acids are also released into the bloodstream. If these aren't used up in physical activity, they can end up sticking to artery walls, a process that can lead to heart disease.

Am I stressed?

Although different people can react in very different ways to the same life events, researchers have found that certain experiences are stressful to large numbers of people. This makes it possible for individuals to get a reasonable idea of how stressed they are and the likelihood of suffering health problems as a result.

Look down the list on pages 136–8 and add up the scores for the major life-events you have experienced during the past year. As you'll see, both pleasant and unpleasant events can prove stressful: that's because virtually any significant change can feel unsettling. A total score of 300 or more suggests that you have experienced high levels of stress and that this could affect your health.

I'm stressed out—how can I change?

○ Assess your stress.

Key tips:
➲ Accept that you might be experiencing negative stress. If you're the kind of guy who likes to pretend he's so cool he's practically frozen, you might find it hard to admit you're stressed even to yourself. It might not feel very manly to accept you can't cope, but being honest with yourself could actually require a lot more courage than simply continuing to suppress the truth.
➲ Work out whether you're too stressed. This might not be as obvious as it seems since many of us have lived with stress for so long that it's actually begun to feel almost normal. A good clue is whether you have any of the physical or emotional symptoms of stress (see page 133) or whether you've experienced several significant life event stresses in the past year (see table below).
➲ Work out what's stressing you. In some cases, this will be obvious—you're unhappy at work, you've just split up with your partner, or your roof's been hit by a meteorite and you can't afford to repair it. If the causes aren't so clear-cut, try keeping a stress diary. Every day for a week, note the times when you feel stressed and the symptoms. Then add what you were doing and thinking during, and just before you developed, the symptoms. At the end of the week, look for patterns. What sort of events or thoughts triggered your stress? Getting bills through the post? Using a particular type of computer program at work? Arguing with your partner about which television programs to watch?

Life-event stressor	Score
Health	
Major injury or illness	64
Moderate injury or illness	39
Major change in your usual type and/or amount of recreation	28
Major dental work	23
Major change in eating habits	23
Major change in sleeping habits	23
Minor injury or illness	17
Work	
Loss of job:	
– laid off from work	59
– fired from work	69
Retirement	48
Change to a new type of work	50
Major business adjustment	47
Demotion	39
Trouble with people under your supervision	34
Change in your work hours	32
Trouble with co-workers	32
Transfer	31
More responsibilities	29
Promotion	29
Trouble with your boss	29
Fewer responsibilities	21
Home and family	
Death	
– of your spouse/partner	113
– of your child	103
– of a parent	90
– of a brother or sister	87
Divorce/irrevocable separation	85
Separation due to relationship problems	70

Life-event stressor	Score
Home and family (cont.)	
Birth of a child	56
Pregnancy	55
Adoption of a child	54
Separation from spouse/partner due to work	54
A relative moving in with you	53
Divorce of your parents	52
Miscarriage or abortion	51
Marriage	50
Major change in health of a family member	50
Marital reconciliation	48
Remarriage of a parent	45
Moving home to a different town or part of the country	39
Child leaving home for reasons	
besides attending college or marriage	38
Spouse/partner changes work	37
Major change in living conditions	37
Child leaving home	
– due to marriage	36
– to attend college	34
Birth of grandchild	34
In-law problems	33
Moving home within the same town or city	21
Change in family get-togethers	20
Personal and social	
Being held in jail	71
Death of a close friend	64
Major decision regarding your future	46
Sexual difficulties	44
Engagement to marry	42
'Falling out' of a close personal relationship	41
An accident	38
Beginning or ending school or college	35

Life-event stressor	Score
Personal and social (cont.)	
Girlfriend or boyfriend problems	34
New relationship	34
Major personal achievement	33
Change of school or college	31
Change in religious beliefs	27
Christmas	25
Change in social activities	24
Change in personal habits	24
Change in political beliefs	21
Vacation	20
Minor violation of the law	19
Financial	
Foreclosure on a mortgage or loan	51
Decreased income	49
Investment or credit difficulties	46
Loss or damage of personal property	35
Major purchase	33
Increased income	30
Moderate purchase	18

○ Be tough on the causes of stress. The most permanent solution—but often the hardest—is to eliminate whatever's causing the problem. If your computer keeps crashing, for example, consider dumping it or buying new software. If your neighbor's loud music winds you up when you're trying to relax in the evening, ask them to turn it down. If you can't cope with the amount of work your boss gives you, say 'no' next time you're asked to produce another major report in two days. Since tackling the causes of stress often involves being direct and up front with other people, it could help if you sharpen up your assertiveness skills (see page 121).

○ Improve your ability to cope with stress. It isn't always possible to eliminate all the causes of stress—you can't make the trains run on time when you're late for work, for example, and you can't stop it raining on the day you decide to take your children out for a walk in the country—so it could help if you learnt some ways of managing your stress better.

Key tips:

➲ Talk about it, not to yourself but to friends, family, and colleagues. Simply discussing a problem can make it feel more manageable, and other people can often give you advice or information that actually helps solve it.

➲ Improve your skills. If you find it hard to set clear priorities at work (or anywhere else), take effective time management much more seriously (see page 141). If you dread making presentations at work, go on a training course. If you're getting frustrated surfing for information on the Internet, research more efficient methods of searching. If your dog won't stop chewing your armchair, find out how you can get it to chase the cat instead. Knowing more about how to tackle the problems you face can make a big difference to your stress levels.

➲ Exercise more. When you're stressed, your body is ready for action. You don't have to pretend you're running away from a dinosaur, but some regular moderate or vigorous exercise will help neutralize the adrenaline that's coursing through your veins. One study of 100 workers, 50 of whom exercised regularly and 50 of whom didn't, found that the exercisers had lower levels of stress and felt happier in their work.

➲ Relax more. This doesn't just mean watching extra television. 'Active relaxation' is a much better stressbuster—and isn't a contradiction in terms. Try these two simple exercises for 10 minutes a day and whenever you feel particularly stressed out:

  ○ Tense and relax each of your muscle groups in turn, starting with your feet and then moving up your body. Clench each set of muscles for a few seconds, focus on the feeling and then gradually relax. Finish with your forehead. This exercise helps counteract the muscle tension that accompanies stress.

  ○ Breathe deeply and slowly. One way of making sure your breaths are deep enough is to place a hand on your abdomen (around your navel). That's the area that should be moving in and out, not your chest. You should aim to reduce your relaxed breathing rate to under 10 breaths a minute, although anything under 15 is good. This exercise helps tackle the fast and shallow breathing that occurs when you're feeling stressed.

➲ Try a massage. There's increasing evidence that the techniques of stroking, kneading, and friction effectively stretch and relax muscles. Moreover, your time on the massage table is in a calm space, free from distractions.

(139)

➲ Change your diet.

   ○ Cut down on caffeine (in tea, coffee, and cola drinks)—its effects can easily exacerbate the symptoms of stress. One study found that drinking four or five cups of coffee throughout the morning produces, on average, a 32 per cent rise in adrenaline levels and that these levels remain high until bedtime, even if no caffeine is consumed after 1pm.

   ○ It's also important to avoid foods containing processed carbohydrates or added sugar (e.g. white bread, white pasta, chocolate, biscuits, cakes, etc.). Because these have only a short-term impact on your blood-sugar levels—the levels rise soon after eating but then quickly fall—your body can react by generating an adrenaline boost to keep your muscles going, worsening the effects of any stress.

   ○ Your best bet is to eat more complex and slower-to-digest carbohydrates (e.g. brown rice, brown pasta, wholemeal bread, and plenty of fresh fruit and vegetables).

➲ Learn to meditate. Clinical trials show that regular meditation slows the pulse rate, lowers blood pressure, and reduces the level of stress hormones whizzing around your body. Studies of 'skin resistance'—when someone is relaxed, their skin tends to resist electric current—suggest that it can rise by up to 40 per cent during meditation.

➲ Learn autogenic training. This is a technique that uses specific mental exercises to switch off the body's stress response, with the aim of enabling the body to reach an altered state of consciousness known as 'passive concentration'. Although the technique has to be learnt in special classes and requires considerable practice, it can produce metabolic and brain-wave changes similar to those achieved through meditation.

➲ Try yoga. You don't need to be able to hold your breath for 10 minutes or to dangle your intestines into a running stream to benefit from this well-established stressbusting technique. The movements and stretches improve the circulation and release tension in the muscles.

➲ Get some counseling. Stress can sometimes be exacerbated by unhelpful beliefs or behaviors that are difficult to tackle without expert help. Some people are perfectionists, for example, and become very anxious if there's the slightest defect in anything they do. Others worry too much about letting people down, even if this puts them under intolerable pressure. A third group can feel panicked at the first sign of stress; this in turn increases their stress, creating more panic, and so on in a vicious circle. A counselor can help identify the source of stress and better ways of responding to it.

YOUR BETTER TIME-MANAGEMENT GUIDE

○ Analyze how you spend your time each day and identify where, when, and how you waste it. For example, do you decide to start something but then procrastinate and spend time on irrelevant tasks? Do you allow social calls to interrupt your working day? Do you spend ages looking for telephone numbers or addresses because you don't keep them in one place? Once you've identified the problems, devise solutions. You could, for instance, make a conscious effort to implement your decisions without allowing yourself to be distracted, tell your friends and relatives to call you only in the evenings, and organize a contacts book or database on your computer.

○ At the start of each day, draw up a list of tasks you need to complete. Then rank them in order of priority. (You can repeat the same exercise for your longer-term tasks on a weekly, monthly, or even annual basis).

○ Train yourself to tackle your priority tasks even if you really don't feel like it. One common reason why we put off tasks is that we're worried about the possible consequences. You might be able to get round this in two ways:

➲ Imagine the worst thing that could possibly happen. Perhaps you fear your boss might laugh in your face if you ask for a pay rise or that the bank might withdraw your overdraft altogether if you ask for the limit to be doubled again. Once you've got a vision of your nightmare scenario, ask yourself about the likelihood of it actually happening. The chances are you'll realize that it's very unlikely to occur.

➲ Another strategy—and one that's essentially the opposite of the first—is simply to imagine yourself effortlessly completing the task you're avoiding. So before you march into your boss's office, think about how confident you'll sound when you ask for a rise, how your boss will say you're the best worker in the department, and how you'll be offered at least another five thousand a year. It probably won't happen like that in reality, of course, but the fantasy could still help you to generate enough confidence to do what's needed.

○ Whenever a piece of paper arrives—whether it's the electricity bill at home or a document at work—make an immediate decision about it. If it needs attention, add it to your list of priorities; if you just need to keep it, file it away; if you don't need it, bin it. If you leave it lying around you'll end up looking at it ten times more often than is actually necessary.

YOUR BETTER TIME-MANAGEMENT GUIDE

○ Complete jobs rather than leaving them part-done. You'll almost certainly get something done more quickly if you give it your full attention rather than flitting from task to task.

○ If you're working on something that requires serious concentration, block out as many interruptions as you can. Switch on your answering machine and tell your colleagues or family you don't want to be disturbed unless World War III breaks out.

○ Delegate wherever possible. At work, this may be to colleagues; at home, this could be to your partner, children, or hired help (e.g. you could employ a decorator or a window cleaner to free up more time for yourself).

○ Build breaks into your schedule. You're not a machine (even if you'd like to be)—you need refreshment and rest. Make sure you take a lunchbreak and have time to eat before an evening meeting.

What's stopping you?

I find it hard to relax when I'm feeling stressed

It's a familiar feeling: you've had a hard day at work, your train was delayed, it was pouring with rain but you forgot your umbrella, and, when you finally arrive home and open the front door, you find the dog's pooped on the carpet. You feel like strangling the hound, not settling down for a peaceful evening of yoga or meditation. You also know that even if you tried to relax, your mind would still be churning over the events of the day. Before you reach for the whiskey bottle, you need to know that there are many different ways of relaxing. In other words, relaxation isn't just about having hot baths scented with aromatherapy oils or practicing deep breathing. It can also be about getting physical, such as going for a run, a workout at the gym, a long walk, or dancing. Exercise of almost any sort can help relax your body and your mind.

If I wasn't stressed I'd be bored

Without some level of stress you probably would be bored. (The reverse is also true: prolonged boredom can eventually feel stressful.) But your choice of emotional states doesn't have to be limited to stress or boredom. A state of relaxation, for example, might sound as if it would be boring, but if you're able to achieve it, it probably won't feel like that. It's also possible that you seek out stressful experiences because, although they might feel unpleasant at times, they're less unpleasant than other feelings they distract you from. These uncomfortable feelings could include boredom but also anger, guilt, sadness, shame, or loneliness. If this could be true for you, it might be helpful to ease up on the stress so that you can begin to uncover the feelings it's hiding. You can then decide whether, and how, you want to tackle the underlying problem.

I'm too busy to change

This is a tough one because it can feel as if you're trapped in a vicious circle with no obvious way out. Let's say you're a self-employed accountant. Because you're worried about making enough money, you feel you can't turn work down and you're working long hours. Your partner's starting to complain about the fact that you never seem to be at home. You're feeling increasingly stressed out and you're finding it harder to sleep and concentrate, increasing the pressures you're experiencing at work and requiring you to work even longer hours to clear your desk.

While you can probably carry on like this for some time, eventually you'll reach a point where your life will end up collapsing around you. You could fall ill, your partner could dump you, or you could start making mistakes that will result in your clients taking their accounts elsewhere. Whatever happens, the eventual result is the same: your income will suffer, even though that's the very thing all the hours of extra work were supposed to avoid. Your best option is clearly to act now to prevent possible disaster by limiting your hours of work and ensuring that you spend more time with your partner. You could also look at how you can improve your time management to ensure you're as productive as possible when you're at work.

HOW NOT TO COPE WITH STRESS

These are common responses to stress and may even seem to work in the short term. In the longer-term, however, they're worse than useless.

- Denying there's a problem.
- Drinking too much tea or coffee.
- Smoking cigarettes.
- Using illegal drugs.
- Working very long hours.
- Driving too fast.
- Paying for sex.
- Drinking too much alcohol.
- Comfort eating.
- Watching television undiscriminatingly and excessively.
- Gambling.
- Looking at pornography.

Post-traumatic stress

You're walking home late at night when you hear someone's footsteps close behind you. There are few people about and you nervously quicken your pace. Two seconds later you feel a hand on your shoulder and you're being pushed into an alleyway. You look down and see a huge knife against your stomach; you look up and see two manic eyes staring straight into yours. Completely terrified, you hand over your wallet and beg not to be hurt. You're pushed to the ground and your assailant runs off. You're physically uninjured but it was the most frightening experience of your life.

You're back at work the next day, and although you're a bit tense, you feel all right. In fact, you begin to forget all about it. But then, about three weeks later, you start having nightmares. You're back in that alley ... there's that knife ... you're about to be stabbed ... you panic ... you wake up in a cold sweat. Then you start having flashbacks during the day, too. You find it harder to concentrate. You find you're increasingly scared to walk anywhere, especially at night. It's almost as if you're stuck in time, back when the accident happened.

You're probably suffering from post-traumatic stress disorder (PTSD). Although previously described as 'shell shock' or 'combat fatigue,' it's a condition that doesn't affect just war veterans or survivors of major disasters. Road accidents and crime are common causes, and a survey of almost 6000 Americans found nearly eight per cent have suffered from PTSD at some time in their lives. The symptoms often include flashbacks, nightmares, and obsessively thinking about what happened. If you think you could be suffering from PTSD, see your doctor. You'll probably be referred to a psychiatrist who may use therapy to tackle the unwanted thoughts and give you a sense of control rather than vulnerability, or may prescribe anti-depressants to reduce the anxiety.

THINGS YOU DIDN'T KNOW ABOUT STRESS

○ Sniffing chocolate can help you relax, according to research from Middlesex University in the UK. In laboratory tests, volunteers sat in a 'low-odor' room wearing blindfolds and ear muffles while boffins waved a range of foods under their noses and measured their brain waves. Only chocolate acted as a relaxant. Strawberries, on the other hand, had a stimulating effect on the brain.

○ Try some heavy petting. Recent research suggests that interacting with pets can have a definite relaxing effect. It's not just down to the exercise involved in taking a dog for a walk: even spending time watching ornamental fish can reduce stress, although stroking an animal has been shown to provide the greatest stressbusting benefits.

○ Play it again, man. Listening to music can not only reduce stress but also improve performance under pressure, according to a study of 50 male surgeons. When asked to complete a task, the surgeons were more relaxed, and performed best, when they listened to music of their choosing. They were also more relaxed, and performed better, when listening to the researchers' choice of music than to no music at all.

○ Have a laugh. Humor may inoculate you against stress, suggests a study of students asked to give anxiety-inducing impromptu speeches. Those who spoke after viewing a television comedy show experienced an average increase in heart rate from 70 beats a minute to around 85. But those who spoke without having first seen the show found that their heart rate went up to 100 while speaking.

CHAPTER 11

JOBS FOR THE BOYS:
FINDING WORK THAT WORKS

M en's relationship with work is changing. Just 30 years ago, most men expected to be in a secure and steady job until retirement. If they gave any thought to their health at work, their main concerns probably would have been about avoiding an accident like a girder falling on their head or knowing how to escape if there was a fire. The 21st-century worker finds himself in a very different environment. The massive growth in white-collar work, together with the rapid spread of short-term contracts and the introduction of new technologies, means he's now more likely to be worried about health problems like stress and the hazards of sitting in front of a computer for eight hours a day. With men also increasingly torn between the ever-growing demands of the workplace and the desire to enjoy good relationships with a partner, children, and friends, it should come as no surprise that over 40 per cent of men aged 25–50 believe work has adversely affected their health, according to research by the British Heart Foundation.

But many men still find it hard to look after their health at work. That's partly because they're frightened of losing their jobs in an ever-more competitive labor market, but it's probably also because they just don't think it's very manly to complain about the noise levels, the heat, the stress, or the long hours. When hard-bitten oil-rig owner Harry Stamper, played by Bruce Willis in the film *Armageddon*, is asked by NASA to fly to, and then destroy, a giant asteroid that's on a collision course with the earth, he doesn't refuse to go because he's worried about breathing in some dust; he doesn't ask to be flown home at the end of an eight-hour shift either. For Mr. Stamper, as well as for a large number of other men at work, it's simply a case of when the going gets tough, the tough get going. But it doesn't have to be like this: 'work' and 'good health' still have the potential to become as synonymous as Bruce Willis and absurd movie plots.

Why bother making work healthier?

○ You'll feel less stressed. Eliminating the causes of stress, and finding ways of coping with it better, could help make work more interesting and enjoyable. You'll also be much less likely to drop dead with a heart attack.

○ You'll have more time for the rest of your life. If you can limit your working hours and take your full holiday entitlement, your life could feel much more balanced.

○ You'll protect the only software that really matters. Yes, it *is* possible to leave work without feeling exhausted or suffering from backache, a headache, or eyestrain. You're also much less likely to be injured in an accident or be exposed to toxic substances.

○ You'll become more employable. Making the changes that will improve your health at work could also significantly increase your skills and abilities.

○ You'll enjoy greater job satisfaction. You can't be truly healthy at work if you're bored and unfulfilled; a healthy worker is much more likely to be a happy worker.

○ You'll probably live longer. Unhealthy work often means an unhealthy, and shorter, life.

What is a healthy workplace?

The truly healthy workplace probably doesn't yet exist in reality. If one did, however, it would pay full attention to both the physical and psychological needs of staff at all levels. If you worked there, you'd notice that its key features included:

○ Stringent controls to eliminate the risk of exposure to any toxic substances, including tobacco smoke, and excessive noise levels.

○ Safe systems of work that minimize the risk of accidents as well as longer-term injuries such as muscle and tendon inflammation caused by repetitive movements or backache caused by spending long periods in one position.

○ A well-lit, well-ventilated, temperature-controlled, spacious, and esthetically attractive working environment.

○ Effective stress management, designed both to eliminate the causes of stress and to help you manage stress better.

○ Regular breaks throughout the working day and no requirement for you to work for longer than your contracted hours.

○ Work that creates a sense of responsibility and feels varied, challenging, worthwhile, and under your control.

THE SCIENCE BIT

○ The more hours you work, the worse your health is likely to be, according to an analysis of over 30 separate studies. The problems caused include stress, fatigue, headaches, insomnia, accidents, depression, and heart disease. There's also good evidence that long working hours are associated with increased rates of smoking and drinking as well as a poorer diet and lower levels of exercise.

○ Almost 90 per cent of managers believe stress is having an adverse effect on their health, morale, work effectiveness, and relationships, according to a survey by the UK Institute of Management. (Ninety per cent of those questioned were men.) Most are experiencing physical symptoms attributable to stress, particularly difficulties sleeping and feeling constantly irritable or impatient.

○ Almost three quarters of working men report difficulties managing work and family obligations, according to a survey of working people in Ohio. When asked to choose between work and home life, 90 per cent of men said they were happier and more 'fulfilled as a person' when at home. Unsurprisingly, 55 per cent would like to work fewer hours.

○ A lack of control over work is a major cause of health problems, according to a long-term study of over 17,000 British male civil servants. Employees in the lowest grades—such as messengers and office support staff—are three times more likely to die within a given time period than the senior administrators. A low-grade job is actually a stronger predictor of premature death from heart disease than smoking, obesity, and high blood pressure. The key factor is stress, a problem that affects the lowest grade staff most because they have least control over their jobs, are much more likely to be bored, and have little opportunity to develop or use new skills.

○ Men threatened with job insecurity are more likely to experience health problems, put on weight, and develop narrowed arteries than men in secure employment, according to a large British study.

○ Unemployment is bad for health too. Unemployed men are more likely to die prematurely, particularly from suicide and lung cancer. In fact, the excess death rate among unemployed men could be at least 20 per cent.

○ Training that enables you to do the job as well as improve your long-term employability.
○ A culture that encourages co-operation and equal opportunities for all, and which strives to eliminate discrimination and bullying.
○ A management structure that is open and in which you and other staff at all levels can participate.
○ Contracts of employment that help you to feel valued and loyal to the organization. You'd be entitled to sufficient job security and pay as well as family-friendly policies, including a right to paid paternity and parental leave.

Your current work probably contains very few (if any) of these important characteristics. But even if your employer's concern for your health and well-being extends little beyond hoping you feel well enough to turn up for work, you can still take steps to ensure that the seven, eight, or ten hours you spend at work each day are as healthy as you can make them.

My job is killing me—how can I change?

○ Take more interest in health and safety at work. Most of us worry more about our next pay increase than we do about leaving work every day feeling as if we've spent it in boot camp. There are now regulations controlling many workplace hazards, from exposure to asbestos to the length of time that can be spent using a computer. If you don't know what the rules are, and how to get them enforced, find out. One of the best sources of information is your trade union. (If you're not a member, consider joining—it's probably the best means you've got of persuading your firm to take its health and safety responsibilities seriously).
○ Spend less time at work. Sometimes you have no choice but to stay late in order to get the job done; at other times, you might be reluctant to leave when you've done your contracted hours, or even to take your full holiday entitlement, because you're worried your boss will mark you down as a slacker. (This increasingly common phenomenon has been aptly described as 'presenteeism').

Key tips:
➲ Accept that staying at work when you're feeling exhausted and resentful, or when your mind is on what you'd rather be doing, isn't productive.
➲ If you need to justify going home on time to yourself, remember all the extra unpaid hours you've worked in the past—haven't you already exceeded the call of duty?

➲ Remember that workers with more balanced lives—who make time for relationships, cultural activities, travel, exercise, hobbies, and volunteering—are often much more productive. They not only feel fresher at work but also have a range of other experiences to draw on.

➲ If you seem to have too much to do in a normal working day, try to improve your time management (see page 141).

➲ Focus on producing high-quality work on time rather than on merely spending time at work. Let your employer judge you by your outputs, not your inputs.

➲ If you can't go home because you're a 'workaholic'—in other words, if you find it hard to stop working or thinking about work—then you may need to do more to get your life back into balance.

   ○ Think about why you've allowed work to occupy a disproportionately significant place in your life. What gap is it filling (e.g. does it make you feel valued or important)? Is it a means of distracting you from other problems?

   ○ Reflect on the consequences of being a workaholic. It could be making you very one-dimensional, for instance, or be damaging your relationships with others.

   ○ If you decide you want to change, it may help if you fix a limit to your working hours. When your time's up, you go home, however wrong it might feel. It's also worth getting support, perhaps from a partner or a friend, to help you stick to your decision. (For more information about tackling any addiction, including work, see pages 97–100.)

➲ Think flexibly about how you can create more time and opportunities for your life outside of work. Working more from home using new technology (so-called 'teleworking') could save you commuting time and enable you to be more productive. If you can afford to do it, part-time work or job-sharing might enable you to pursue more leisure interests or take up volunteering. Negotiating a long period of sabbatical leave from work might provide the opportunity to complete a long-cherished project.

○ Take regular breaks throughout the day. The lunch break may be becoming as anachronistic as typewriters and carbon paper, but there's little doubt that, for most of us, a mid-day break is a great energizer.

○ Tackle your stress. Eliminating the causes of stress is the best option, but, because this isn't always possible, it's also important to find ways of coping better. Relaxation techniques, massage, exercise, and changing your diet can all help (see Chapter 10).

COMPUTER SAFETY

Sure, you can write very important reports, surf the Internet, and play *Tomb Raider*—but do you know how to do all that for eight hours a day, five days a weeks, and still feel like a human being? If not, here's your complete computer-survival guide.

Dangers

Back	Back pain.
Arms	Repetitive Strain Injury (RSI)—typically pain in fingers, wrists, arms, or shoulders; tenderness; swelling; can become chronic if not treated early.
Eyes	Sore eyes, eyestrain, blurred vision.
Brain	Headaches, tiredness, nausea, stress, irritability. In longer term, anxiety, stomach problems, depression, high blood pressure.
Skin	Rashes. Symptoms often appear within four hours of starting work and disappear overnight.

Possible causes

Back	Poor back support; no feet support; seat too low or high; keyboard and/or screen at the wrong height; posture twisted because computer screen at wrong angle.
Arms	Rapid, repetitive movements; stress; poor posture; poorly designed workstation, especially bad keyboard.
Eyes	Spending too much time using computer; images difficult to read; glare on screen, bad lighting; screen too small.
Brain	Repetitive, boring work; unrealistic deadlines; long hours; inadequate software or hardware problems; poor training; too much background noise. Ozone from laser printers can cause headaches and nausea, also eye and nose irritation.
Skin	Combination of over-dry atmosphere, inadequate ventilation, the heat of the screen and excessive static electricity.

COMPUTER SAFETY

What to do

Back Use a chair with adjustable seat height, backrest, and seat tilt; sit upright with both feet on floor or footrest and seat sloping slightly down; position VDU so you are facing it directly but also looking slightly down at it; use a document holder to minimize neck movements; go for a walk; if your back gets stiff, exercise it.

Arms Use a desk and chair with adjustable seat heights (when working, your elbows should be bent at 90 degrees); avoid portable computers; keep a soft touch on the keys; don't overuse the cursor (use Page Up/Down keys rather than scrolling); consider getting an ergonomic keyboard. If you have RSI, rest until you're better; see a doctor or physiotherapist.

Eyes Have an eye test; adjust the contrast or brightness; make sure you have a fully adjustable screen with large enough characters; change the screen color combination; fit an anti-glare filter; position the screen at right angles to windows and at about arm's length from your eyes; exercise the eyes by regularly focusing on distant objects; proof-read on paper, not on the screen.

Brain Ensure working environment—noise, light, furniture—is suitable (acoustic screens can reduce noise); vary your workload; get proper training for the software you're using; position laser printers in separate, well-ventilated areas; learn how to relax—don't smoke or drink more to cope.

Skin Install humidifiers and plants; improve ventilation; reduce the electrostatic charge (natural fabrics in the office will help).

Every part of your body will benefit if you take regular breaks (spend no longer than 50 minutes in every hour at your computer).

COMPUTER SAFETY

The following six stretching exercises will also benefit anyone who spends long periods in a fixed position. All these can be done while sitting upright in your chair, so you don't need to worry about having to jump up and down in the middle of your workplace.

○ Lateral neck rotations. Keeping your head upright and your body stationary, with your arms hanging by your side, turn your head to the left and hold for five seconds. Now turn your head through to the right and hold for five seconds. Repeat twice more.

○ Shoulder shrugs. Look to the front and let your arms hang by your side. Shrug your shoulders up and hold for five seconds before lowering. Repeat twice more.

○ Seated calf raises. Place both feet flat on the floor about six inches apart. Leaving your toes on the floor, lift up both heels as far as you can. Hold for five seconds and repeat twice more.

○ Resisted arm curls. Rest your right hand on your right thigh and place your left hand on your right wrist. Then push down with your left hand and up with your right arm. Hold for five seconds and repeat twice more. Then repeat again for the other side.

○ Wrist rolling. Let your arms hang by your side. Keeping your arms still, lift your fingers until your hands are pointing away from you on either side with the palms facing the floor. Hold for five seconds and then curl your hands in so that your fingers are pointing up toward your armpits. Hold for five seconds. Repeat twice more.

○ Back stretch. Place both hands lightly on the top of your head and bend backward over the backrest of the chair. Hold for five seconds and repeat twice more.

DELIVER US FROM E-MAIL

Some people now find over 100 e-mail messages waiting for them when they arrive for work each day, and they are constantly interrupted by incoming mail. This volume of mail can quickly become a source of stress and mental fatigue.

Key tips:
- ➲ Don't open mail that is obviously advertising—delete it immediately.
- ➲ Switch off your e-mail alert—you can then prevent interruptions and discipline yourself to check your mail just two or three times a day.
- ➲ Don't acknowledge receipt of all your messages—reply only when strictly necessary.
- ➲ Unsubscribe yourself from useless Internet discussion groups.
- ➲ Don't send unnecessary e-mail (that includes copying messages to people who don't really need to see them)—it'll only generate more replies.

○ Get support. Developing your social networks in the workplace could help protect you against some of the consequences of stress by providing an opportunity for you to talk about your problems. You can also work with colleagues to suggest practical changes that will make the workplace healthier. Self-employed workers can often get similar support through professional associations.

○ Learn to love change. Like it or not, you're going to have to if you want to keep your stress levels under control. There's no longer such a thing as 'the job for life' in any sector or profession. Almost any individual has to be prepared to move around between employers and perhaps accept periods of freelance work. It's no longer realistic to think of a career that consists of regular promotions until you're given a key to the executive washroom.

○ Seek out learning and training opportunities. If you know how to do your job better, it will probably feel more under your control, less stressful, and more rewarding. As you become more skilled, you'll also become more employable.

Key tips:
- ➲ Understand that the 'shelf-life' of current knowledge and skills is getting ever shorter. There's no way you'll survive in the emerging job market if you think education is a one-stop shop which ended when you left school or college. The new buzzwords are 'lifelong learning'.

BEATING THE BULLY

Bullying affects the workplace as much as the school playground: about 50 per cent of people say they have experienced bullying at some stage in their working lives, and over 75 per cent say they've witnessed it. Men and women are bullied in equal numbers. It affects not only victims' job satisfaction, work performance, and career development but also results in classic stress-related symptoms such as headaches, insomnia, skin complaints, ulcers, depression, and even suicide.

If you're being bullied:
- Try to stand firm: tell the bully you won't tolerate personal remarks.
- Avoid being alone with the bully.
- Ask colleagues if they're having similar problems.
- Keep a record of all incidents.
- Discuss the problem with your trade-union representative or personnel department.
- Consider making a formal complaint.

⮑ Don't think about training solely in terms of increasing your technical competence, vital though that is. Modern employers are increasingly looking for a wider set of less tangible skills, especially strategic thinking, self-management, team-working, awareness of other cultures, and 'emotional intelligence'—in other words, being good at communicating, negotiating, and inspiring others. You can't wake up in the morning with these abilities—they need to be learnt through training and a commitment to personal change. Since men's upbringing can mean that many of these skills are often harder for them to acquire than for women, some organizations are beginning to introduce 'men's development' programs. Don't worry: these don't involve drumming sessions, running naked through the woods, or eating loads of rice cakes and lentils. Rather, they focus on exploring issues like male identity and relationships with women as well as providing men with an opportunity to enhance their interpersonal skills.

- Consider more radical solutions. Most men have been brought up to believe it's their role in life to get the 'best' (i.e. highest paid and/or most prestigious and powerful) job they can. It's not surprising, therefore, that we often end up in jobs

COMPUTERPHOBIA

Computers are now an integral part of virtually every workplace but between a quarter and one-third of us are anxious about using them to some degree, while one in twenty have severe symptoms, including sweaty palms, palpitations, and even panic attacks. These problems are usually caused by poor training, which has left the computerphobe afraid of looking foolish or feeling humiliated whenever he makes a mistake.

For once, self-help isn't the answer—encountering unexpected problems with no available assistance can simply reinforce feelings of anxiety. Computerphobes seem to learn best in groups, which not only provide lots of encouragement but also focus on how to overcome potential problems. People with the highest levels of anxiety can also benefit from a process of 'desensitization'—in other words, slowly increasing levels of exposure to computers—in the same way as others might be helped to overcome a fear of spiders or flying.

we don't really value (or which don't value us), working long hours, and feeling that being made redundant represents personal failure. In order to create a life in which work creates a sense of fulfillment and satisfaction, we may need to change the way we think about it as well as the way we do it.

Key tips:
➲ Ask yourself what you consider the true purpose of your life to be. One way to think about this is to imagine lying on your deathbed asking yourself whether your work truly reflected your deepest needs and values. Will you look back and feel content with your ceaseless efforts to increase your income or will you be left with regrets that this meant you chose to sacrifice your long-held desire to become an artist or to do the kind of work that would help create the sort of society you'd like to see?
➲ Consider whether you can transform the work you already do to reflect your goals or whether you need to look for a different job or even a different form of employment (e.g. self-employment).
➲ Be prepared to take a risk. Your ability to attempt any dramatic change may well depend on your personal circumstances—it may be that you'll have to wait until your children have left school, for example, or you've paid off college loans—but one thing is clear: in the long run, it can be more painful

carrying on as you are than taking a risk and doing the kind of work that meets your real needs.

Coping with unemployment

Most men find losing a job a stressful and demeaning experience. Not only is there a big drop in their standard of living but they can also experience an even larger fall in status and self-worth. And there are all those extra hours to fill. There's no easy way of dealing with unemployment, but it is possible to do more than sit at home watching endless repeats on daytime television.

Key tips:
- ⮞ Accept that losing your job probably isn't your fault (unless you embezzled the firm's pension fund). You can't blame yourself for the inevitable slumps in the economic cycle.
- ⮞ Get all the advice and support you can to help you find another job. Seeing a careers counselor is an option, especially if you'd like to change direction.
- ⮞ Consider how you can spend time creatively (and without spending much money). Exercise is a good option: brisk walking or jogging are nil-cost possibilities.
- ⮞ If you have young children, you could see unemployment as an opportunity to play a larger role in their upbringing.
- ⮞ Spend time with friends. It's vital not to become isolated when you're unemployed, and you may well need people to talk to about your situation.
- ⮞ Try volunteering. It's inherently worthwhile, an excellent way to meet new people, and can even increase your work skills. It might even prolong your life. A study of over 1200 Americans found that those doing up to 40 hours voluntary work a year were about three times less likely to die over a seven-and-a-half year period than those who didn't. It probably protects health by providing a sense of purpose and meaning.

What's stopping you?

Many of my colleagues smoke and I'm worried about the effects on my health, but I don't want to seem a wimp by complaining
  Would you feel a wimp if you complained about someone who kicked you every time they passed? Probably not, yet your inhalation of your colleagues' smoke could be causing you far greater long-term damage. One study found that exposure

at work increases the risk of lung cancer by almost 40 per cent. This is a workplace health and safety issue, not an argument between you and your colleagues, and you should ask your employer to introduce a workplace smoking ban. It may well feel embarrassing to raise the issue, but you'd also be taking a courageous step which could ultimately benefit everybody who works in your company.

I almost always work at least 50 or 60 hours a week and hardly ever see my children. The thing is, I love my work, too, and can't seem to spend less time at the office

There's no law that says you have to spend more time with your family if you don't want to but you should consider the possible long-term consequences of being a so-called 'absent father'. Your children may grow increasingly distant from you and find it hard to feel comfortable with you when you are at home. They may even feel start to feel angry with you, especially if they see that your absence is making their mother unhappy.

If you decide you would like to spend more time with your children, consider how you could reduce your working hours without losing the satisfaction you derive from work. Better time management might help, for example, as could being more assertive about refusing extra work. You might also want to consider whether you are spending more time at work because you find home life stressful, perhaps because you have relationship problems with your partner or you are uncertain how to interact with your children. If this is the case, in the long run you might be better off tackling these problems rather than avoiding them. There are relationship-counseling organizations and fathers' groups that could help.

THINGS YOU DIDN'T KNOW ABOUT WORK AND HEALTH

○ Driving on business is a serious occupational hazard. In fact, people who drive 25,000 miles a year as part of their job are at the same risk of dying in an accident as a coal miner, according to a research by the UK's Royal Society for the Prevention of Accidents.

○ Sick-building syndrome isn't a malingerer's excuse for a day off work—it really does exist. An estimated 30–50 per cent of new or refurbished buildings are affected, and the symptoms typically include headaches, tiredness, a dry throat, skin problems, dry eyes, muscular aches, and a blocked or runny nose. The causes aren't yet fully understood, but air-conditioned and open-plan offices with furniture and equipment that block the flow of air have been implicated. Problems may also be caused by a chemical reaction between ozone emitted by photocopiers and organic pollutants found in carpets, perfumes, and wood. The result is an irritant chemical which can affect breathing.

○ Colleagues talking, phones ringing, e-mails bleeping, photocopiers whirring—these unexceptional, low-level, everyday sounds can seriously affect productivity and stress levels. They can reduce performance of simple cognitive tasks, like memory and mental arithmetic, by about one third compared to a quiet environment, according to research at Reading University in the UK.

○ Exercise not only reduces stress levels, it also makes you more productive. NASA discovered that staff who worked out were more likely to work at full efficiency all day while other employees' efficiency decreased by 50 per cent in the two hours before going home.

○ Job satisfaction isn't good only for the health of individual workers—it's also good for the economic health of their company. In fact, it's a better predictor of profitability than competitive strategy, market share, or spending on research and development, according to a 10-year study of 42 UK companies. Employees are most likely to be happy when they feel valued and trusted.

CHAPTER 12

THE REALITY OF RELATING:

GETTING THE MOST OUT OF GETTING CLOSE

Relationships are important. Very few of us would choose to live in virtual isolation, without regular contact with a partner, relatives, friends, or work colleagues. Our experience of closeness begins at the moment of conception, and we're unlikely ever to be able to feel completely satisfied and fulfilled without it. Even though men have been criticized for their lack of relationship skills, there's no doubt that things are now improving fast: they're beginning to attach a higher value to relationships and to feel much more comfortable about communicating thoughts and feelings. Millennial Man is much less likely to idolize traditional male heroes like Clint Eastwood, who, in his spaghetti westerns, played the part of a man so isolated he didn't even have a name, let alone a wide circle of friends and a partner with whom he shared his life.

But men can still find relationships difficult. We may struggle to maintain friendships with other men, especially as we get older, while the soaring divorce and separation rates are testimony to the difficulties we face in sustaining long-term, loving relationships with partners. Some men even experience problems with the notion of commitment itself—they may be passionately in love, but they can still find the idea of 'settling down' with a partner about as exciting as spending an evening watching 20-year-old episodes of *Dallas*. Sadly, a survey of over 7000 US men found that 43 per cent haven't found the warmth and closeness in their lives that they want. This matters, not only because it's no fun feeling lonely and isolated but also because the quality of our relationships can profoundly affect our health.

Why bother with relationships?

○ You'll feel better. Humans are social animals, and we're much more likely to feel good about ourselves if we have a rich and diverse network of social contacts. Simply knowing that someone else likes you, enjoys your company, and wants to spend time with you can help you feel valued and significant.
○ You'll look after your health better. Men who have a partner, or a wider range of relationships, generally eat healthier foods and drink and smoke less. They're also more likely to seek medical help if they develop a health problem.
○ You'll be ill less. Relationships strengthen the immune system, reducing susceptibility to a range of minor infections like colds.
○ You'll live longer. The more connections you have with other people, the more likely you are to survive for longer if you do become seriously ill, and the less likely you are to die prematurely from any cause.

Why do relationships matter?

Rates of mental illness, suicide, heart disease, and cancer are all higher among men without partners or good social networks. In fact, it's been calculated that social isolation is a medical risk factor comparable to high blood pressure, obesity, and lack of exercise. Some research even suggests that a lack of social relationships can have as much of a negative impact on health as smoking.

There are several theories about why relationships can make such a difference:
○ Other people can help protect us against the full impact of stressful events. Being able to talk to someone about, for example, an important job interview or the death of a parent can provide an important emotional cushion.
○ A partner or friend can directly affect our health by providing warnings of potentially dangerous behaviors, such as driving too fast, smoking, or drinking excessively. They might also encourage us to visit the doctor at times when we might be tempted to dismiss the stabbing pains in our stomach as too trivial to bother about.
○ Social pressures may make it more likely that we'll follow a doctor's advice, and we're more likely to be able to rest and recuperate if there are other people around to cook us meals, wash our pyjamas, and listen to our moans about how much it hurts.

THE SCIENCE BIT

○ Lonely people tend to have poorer immune systems. A study of 75 medical students at around the time of their final examinations found that those who felt most lonely had significantly lower scores on a key measure of immune function. Other studies show that separated and divorced men also have a weaker immune system, although the impairment tends to be less when it's men who initiate the break-up.

○ Social isolation increases the chances of catching a cold. When 276 healthy volunteers, aged 18–55, were given nasal drops containing a common cold virus, those with richer social networks were less likely to catch a cold. In fact, those with fewest social ties were over four times as susceptible as those with the best social lives.

○ Relationships are related to surviving longer with an illness. Men with prostate cancer who have partners are likely to live longer than those who are divorced, single, separated, or widowed, according to a study of almost 147,000 men in the USA. Men with HIV who have more than average levels of social support are two to three times less likely to develop AIDS than men with below average levels of social support, according to a five-and-a-half year US study.

○ Even the support of strangers can make a difference. Researchers randomly assigned patients who'd had surgery for malignant melanoma (an aggressive type of skin cancer) either to a support group or a comparison group. The support-group patients met for just 90 minutes a week for six weeks but were much more likely to be alive six years later than those who'd attended the comparison group. In fact, three times as many people died after attending the comparison group than the support group.

○ Men with partners are less likely to die prematurely. Single and never-married men are one-and-a-half times more likely to die of heart disease, according to a British study of over 7700 middle-aged men. Men who divorced were almost twice as likely to die from heart disease and four times as likely to die from any other cause.

○ Loneliness is linked to death. A long-term study of almost 7000 people living near San Francisco found that men lacking social and community ties (contact with friends and relatives, marriage, and church and group membership) were more than twice as likely to die during a nine-year period. Those with fewest social connections were at greater risk of dying from heart disease, stroke, cancer, respiratory diseases, gastro-intestinal diseases, and all other causes.

THE SCIENCE BIT

○ The quality of relationships could also matter. A study of over 8450 middle-aged Israeli men found that those who felt their wives provided little love and support were twice as likely to develop a duodenal ulcer as those men whose wives showed their love and support.

I'm a bit of a loner—how can I change?

○ Accept that relationships are important. Although you might believe that men should be independant and free of emotional ties and commitments, or that work is far more important than your social life, ask yourself whether you have the closeness and intimacy in your life that you'd really like. Remember, too, that even icons of masculinity sometimes feel the need for closeness: both Superman and James Bond eventually married (although, regrettably, 007 was widowed later the same day).

○ Review your priorities. If you want to improve your relationships, you may have to give them a higher profile in your life. To get an idea of how significant they are for you at present, try ranking the following 20 priorities. Put the most important at the top and the least important at the bottom.

○ Job satisfaction
○ Many casual sexual partners
○ A close relationship with your children (whether or not you currently have any)
○ Independence
○ Good health
○ A close, loving, and long-term relationship with a partner
○ Close friendships
○ Regular (and great) sex
○ Living in your dream house

○ An active social life
○ Freedom
○ Career progression
○ A muscular body
○ Twice your current income
○ A loving family (parents, siblings, etc.)
○ Being famous
○ The holiday of a lifetime
○ Excelling at your favorite sport
○ Feeling at the center of your community
○ The car you've always wanted

There are no right or wrong answers, but if you want to develop your relationships you might need to think about moving them toward the top of your list. After all, it's

REAL HEALTH FOR MEN

harder to develop a richer social network if you spend most of your time working or if you feel it's more important to own a fantastic car.

○ Since your relationships are unlikely to improve on their own, or by you waiting until the 'right person' happens to turn up (they almost certainly won't), you need to consider taking positive action.

Key tips:
➲ Find ways to meet more people. If you spend all your spare time watching television or surfing the Internet, it's pretty obvious that you're not going to meet any new people. Consider starting an activity that gives you the opportunity to interact socially. The options include joining a gym or an evening class, becoming involved with a political party, or volunteering (e.g. working in a shelter for homeless people or rescuing stray cats).
➲ Take some risks. You can't make friends or start relationships if you don't begin by talking to people. If you find it hard to initiate a conversation with a stranger, ask a mutual friend or colleague to introduce you. If you want to get to know someone better, start by suggesting meeting for lunch or a quick drink after work. Don't wait to be asked first—and don't assume that just because the other person doesn't take the initiative it automatically means that he or she doesn't like you. Remember, too, that it's perfectly normal to fear rejection by someone you're attracted to (sexually or not).
➲ Be the kind of guy people want to know—without having a personality transplant or extensive plastic surgery.
   ○ One of the best ways in which you can appear interesting to other people is simply to be interested in them. Just listening carefully to what they have to say and asking questions about their lives can make a big, big difference.
   ○ Share information about your own life, particularly in terms of your own thoughts and feelings. Giving people an honest account of your experiences can make you seem much more likeable and worth getting to know than if you just drone on about all the countries you've visited on business or the quickest way to drive to work.
   ○ Showing a passionate interest in something—whether it's the movies, books, or astronomy (but maybe not your collection of Action Man dolls)—could help too.
➲ Accept that not everybody will like you, just as you don't like everyone you meet.
➲ Communicate, communicate, communicate. The key to any good relationship, or sorting out a relationship problem, is effective communication.

THE ART OF BETTER COMMUNICATION

No one can accurately guess what you're thinking and feeling: you have to spell it out. And the same goes for you: if you want to know about someone else's experience, you'll have to ask. If two people don't share honest information with each other, there's every likelihood that their relationship will be characterized by misunderstanding and conflict rather than warmth and affection. It is, of course, possible for honest communication to cause its own problems—it may reveal irreconcilable differences, for example—but becoming aware of these sooner rather than later may well be preferable.

Key tips:

⊃ Do more than have a conversation. Discussing whatever interests you—sport, politics, classic cars—is a vital part of any relationship. But there's more to communication that enjoying abstract discussions and arguments. It's about what you feel as well as what you think.

⊃ Be honest about your feelings. If you don't say what you really mean, or don't say anything at all, the other person can't respond in any effective way. For example, your partner's malodorous breath may make kissing unpleasant, but if you don't mention it nothing can change. You might feel like backing off because you don't want to hurt your partner's feelings, but this will just leave you unhappy and could start causing bigger problems (your partner might even start thinking you're falling out of love). If you're up front, the problem can then be much more easily solved.

⊃ Listen to what the other person says. If you make assumptions, you'll probably get it wrong. If you interrupt, try to shout someone down, or keep changing the subject, you'll never find out about their perspective. Wait until they've finished before you ask for clarification or give your opinion.

⊃ Accept that the other person's feelings and opinions may be different from your own and that he or she is entitled to them whether or not you like what you hear. It's fine for you to feel upset, but that doesn't make it acceptable for you to try to stop the other person thinking and feeling as they do. Your best option is, in turn, to explain how what they've said makes you feel.

⊃ Treat the other person as an equal. If you believe, or act as if, they're somehow inferior or stupid (or that you are) then you're unlikely to be able to communicate very effectively with them.

THE ART OF BETTER COMMUNICATION

➲ Good communication isn't helped by blaming, criticizing, or insulting the other person. You don't need to be Sigmund Freud to realize that saying 'I'd fancy you more if you weren't so fat' is likely to be much less effective than 'I love you very much and I'd find you even sexier if you were a little bit trimmer.' Being sarcastic or calling your partner an 'idiot' or a 'bitch' isn't likely to improve mutual communication either.

➲ Be assertive. This doesn't mean finding ways of aggressively imposing your views. It means being direct and honest about what you want but also being prepared to negotiate. Your aim should be to try and achieve a compromise in which you and the other person both feel you've got what you want (psychologists call this a 'win-win' outcome). This is preferable to a 'win-lose' outcome which, although it might make the 'victor' feel better for a while, is likely to result in the 'loser' feeling resentful and angry—emotions likely to cause more problems in the future.

➲ Accept you might be wrong. Rather than stubbornly sticking to a position you know is mistaken, be prepared to admit that you could be the one who needs to consider changing some attitudes or behaviors.

➲ Choose your moment. If you've got something difficult to say, it's probably better done in private (not in the middle of a supermarket, for example) and at a time when the other person isn't rushed or stressed. If you're going to tell your partner you're seriously dissatisfied with your sex life, it's probably unwise to do so just before they leave home for a crucial job interview.

➲ Be flexible. If you find it hard to communicate verbally with another person, see if you can agree to have a dialogue by means of exchanging letters. This might provide enough 'emotional space' to enable both of you to say what you want and to be able to reflect on what's being said. You might then find it easier to meet to discuss whatever's going on.

➲ Don't assume women speak a different language, let alone come from another planet. Although men and women often have different communication styles—women tend to focus more on feelings, men more on facts—it's perfectly possible for them to get on the same wavelength with practice.

THE ART OF BETTER COMMUNICATION

➲ Be prepared. Honest communication can create strong emotions—after all, if you tell someone that they've got body odor, that you'd prefer them to drink less, or that you don't love them any more, it's only realistic to expect expressions of grief, resentment, or anger. But if both of you are committed to honest dialogue, there's a very good chance you can reach some sort of resolution. Remember: if things get too heated, you can always ask for a 10-minute truce—one of you can then leave the room to let things cool down before you resume.

○ Be prepared to end relationships that, despite your best efforts, just aren't working. Good relationships make you feel nourished, not depleted, and if you find that you're hanging onto a poor one for old time's sake, guilt, or because you're scared of being on your own, then you should seriously consider whether it's time to be honest with yourself and the other person. Your energies might well be better invested in developing new and satisfying relationships than sticking with ones that have become less salvageable than the *Titanic*.

○ The end of an intimate relationship can be extremely traumatic and difficult to come to terms with. Some men try to deal with it by distracting themselves with work or by numbing themselves with drink or drugs. This strategy might work for a while but can't take away the painful feelings for good; it also isn't very healthy. Dealing with a relationship breakdown is never easy, but there are effective ways of coping better.

Key tips:

➲ Accept that you're probably going to feel bad. Don't try and blot out any feelings of shock, dislocation, loss, or anger because they feel unpleasant or because you believe that, as a man, you should be able to take hard knocks as if they were little worse than gnat bites.

➲ Talk about your feelings to people you trust. You could also keep a journal in which you write your innermost thoughts.

➲ Accept your share of responsibility for the relationship breakdown. Even though you may feel the other person is totally at fault, this is, in fact, unlikely. Changing your perspective could help you come to terms with any anger you feel toward your ex-partner: anger is an emotion that's natural but also corrosive to you in the long-term; a new perspective could also enable you to reflect on your own behavior and make changes that could benefit your future relationships.

➲ Don't rush into another relationship until you've fully mourned the loss of the last one. Although it's tempting to seek out a new partner very quickly, a relationship is unlikely to flourish if it remains overshadowed by the one that went before.

➲ Try not to draw children into battles with your ex-partner. Whatever your feelings about each other you remain co-parents of your children, and your joint responsibility is to provide them with as much love and stability as possible.

○ Seek support. Relationships are hugely complicated. Many of the difficulties we experience with them have their origins in childhood or in previous adult relationships. If your father was a bully, for example, you might well feel cautious about forming friendships with other men; if your mother was over-protective, you might feel trapped when you develop a close relationship with a woman; if you felt abandoned or unloved as a child you might find it harder to commit yourself to relationships. Because it's easy to remain unaware of these deeper psychological processes, they can't always be resolved simply by trying to talk through current problems. It may sometimes be necessary to call on the help of an expert counselor or therapist, especially if a relationship is in crisis. It's possible to see a counselor either on your own or as a couple (or, indeed, as a family unit).

Healthy relationships aren't just with people

PETS

It might sound improbable, but a relationship with a pet (or, as they're increasingly known, 'companion animals'), can provide major health benefits.

○ Male pet owners have significantly lower blood fat and blood pressure levels—both major heart disease risk factors—according to a large Australian study. These findings can't be explained by other factors such as smoking, diet, or body-mass, and are irrespective of the type of pet owned.

○ Pet ownership is one of the best predictors of surviving for more than a year after a heart attack, according to a US study. This isn't due simply to dog owners getting more exercise since other pet owners also benefit.

○ Other research demonstrates that blood pressure falls when stroking a dog, and even the presence of the animal in the room seems to have a calming effect (unless, of course, it's an unmuzzled and angry Rottweiler).

Pets are good for us because we can be openly affectionate toward them, they can make us laugh, comfort us when we're feeling down, and (in the case of dogs) create an incentive to take more exercise. Animals rely on their owners for care and attention, and can therefore enhance our sense of responsibility, purpose, and self-esteem. Pets are an excellent topic of conversation, creating opportunities to develop and deepen social relationships (with other humans, that is). Animal behavior also tends to be predictable, providing a source of stability in an ever-changing, stressful world. You can talk to your pet, confide in it, hug it, or chuck it out into the garden, and—unlike most people—it will remain a constant, unquestioning companion.

THE SPIRITUAL WORLD

Having a relationship with the spiritual world, including God or another religious being, can also be good for your health. One US study of almost 4000 people aged 65 and over found that the higher your level of religious activity, the lower your blood pressure is likely to be. Other research into doctors, African Americans, and elderly hospital and nursing-home patients suggests that participation in religious activity is associated with higher levels of satisfaction with life. There's also evidence that attending religious services boosts key aspects of the immune system.

It's not exactly clear why spiritual belief is good for you. Assuming the health benefits aren't just a deity's way of saying 'thank you,' it could be that believers are more likely to have a healthier lifestyle, that spiritual practices relieve stress, or that the idea that we're somehow part of a 'bigger picture' offers emotional comfort as well as a sense of personal significance. It's also possible that participating in a spiritual community offers access to higher levels of practical and emotional support.

You can't force yourself to adopt a religion or a spiritual outlook just because it might be good for your health. That would be absurd. But it could be worth at least opening your mind to the possibilities of spiritual experiences. We tend to feel more in touch with this non-rational dimension of human life at times when we confront issues of life and death (when a loved one is seriously ill, for example), when witnessing the grandeur of nature, or when experiencing the beauty of a piece of music or a work of art. Feeling a deep connection to another human being, or even an animal, can also create strong spiritual feelings.

RELATIONSHIPS WITH CHILDREN

If you have children, your relationship with them is undoubtedly one of the most important you'll ever have. But although men are now trying hard to become more active and involved parents, many still struggle to become as close to their offspring as they would like. This is particularly true for men who don't live with their children.

Key tips:

➲ Be at the birth. Taking part in this crucial process can help you bond with your new baby. It's good to be well-prepared so you know what to expect and how to help your partner during labor.

➲ Take time off after the birth. Spending time with a new baby is crucial: how else can you get to know him or her from the start? If your employer won't provide paternity leave, take some holiday.

➲ Do the dirty stuff. Don't just play with your child: get stuck in with the cleaning, food preparation, and feeding as well as washing their clothes.

➲ Be prepared to get wet. If you want to focus on 'quality time' rather than 'quantity time', make sure you're there to give junior his or her daily bath.

➲ Do the school run. It's a good opportunity to ask about his or her day. Go to parents' evenings to meet the teachers, and, when necessary, take your child to the doctor. It's important to be involved in every aspect of his or her life.

➲ If you're traveling on business, try to phone your children regularly.

➲ Don't become the distant disciplinarian. That might have been your father's role, but it doesn't have to be yours.

➲ Involve your children in your work. Take them to your workplace occasionally so they get to know where you are all day.

➲ If you're separated from your children because you don't live with their mother, do your best to stick to arrangements for visits, use audio- or videotapes to keep in contact, talk regularly on the phone, and write letters.

➲ Tell your children you love them and give them plenty of appropriate physical affection. This will help make them feel more secure, valued, and comfortable with themselves.

What's stopping you?

I find it hard to make friends these days
What's changed? There could be any number of reasons why you're now finding it tough. The first step is to identify them and then formulate an action plan. If your family is taking up a lot of time—perhaps you're caring for children, a sick partner, or elderly parents—see if you can join a parents' or a carers' group to meet others in a similar situation. If you never seem to meet people who share your values and interests, think about where you can go to stand the best chance of finding like-minded people. It's possible that you're expecting too much from friendships and are ruling out in advance those that seem unlikely to replicate the intimate ones you may have experienced when you were younger. Remember: friendships can exist, and be enjoyed, on many different levels. Finally, perhaps you're either passively waiting for someone else to make the first move or not giving enough of yourself to others. One of the best ways to make a friend is to take the risk of behaving like a friend.

Since my partner left me I've felt unable to start another steady relationship
Perhaps you're not ready yet. It can take a long time to get over the end of a relationship, especially for the partner who was left. It's possible that your self-confidence has plummeted and that you can't believe anyone else will want a relationship with you. You could give your self-esteem a boost by listing all the positive things you have to offer a new partner. It could also be worth taking an honest look at why your partner left you and whether you need to change some of your attitudes and behaviors. The best thing you can do is to talk about how you feel about what happened—perhaps to a friend or a counselor—in order to come to terms with it.

Every time I try and discuss a problem with my partner we end up in a row
You may have to take the initiative and try talking to your partner in a different way. First, you need to review where things are going wrong at the moment. Are you raising problems at the wrong time (at bedtime or just before leaving for work, for instance)? Do you quickly get into blaming your partner or start shouting? Or does your partner start blaming or criticizing you, and in response you become angry and vindictive? Once you've worked out what's stopping effective communication, you need to adopt a new strategy. It's possible that talking about how you feel about the problem might be the best

THINGS YOU DIDN'T KNOW ABOUT RELATIONSHIPS

○ Touch is an important component of most close relationships. Not only do most people enjoy it but there's growing evidence that touch—especially massage—can produce significant health benefits, including stress reduction and relaxation. A daily massage for one month significantly enhanced the immune system functioning of HIV-positive gay men, according to one study; another found that a twice-weekly massage reduced adults' anxiety levels and increased their alertness and ability to perform mathematical calculations.

○ When answering the question 'What is it about women that attracts you the most?', 62 per cent of 776 American men taking part in a survey mentioned 'personality,' making it the most frequently mentioned criterion. Next came 'beauty' (55 per cent), followed by 'sense of humor' (48 per cent), 'smile' (48 per cent), and 'intelligence' (48 per cent).

○ Male advertisers in lonely hearts advertisements are much more likely than female advertisers to say they want a youthful partner (42 per cent versus 25 per cent) or a physically attractive one (44 per cent versus 22 per cent), according to a study of 900 advertisements in four US newspapers. But men are much less forthcoming about their own looks: while 50 per cent of women used terms like 'gorgeous', 'pretty,' or 'curvaceous' only 34 per cent of men used comparable terms such as 'athletic', 'hunk,' or 'handsome'.

○ Men may be attracted to women (and vice versa) for some not-so-obvious reasons. There's increasing evidence that pheromones (hormonal secretions sensed by a specific part of the nose) can have surprising effects on our behavior. When men were asked to rate the attractiveness of women in a Vienna University study, they scored them more highly when they were also inhaling the scent of synthetic vaginal pheromones. Other research has found that 74 per cent of men who used a synthetic male pheromone reported increased sexual interest from women, and when a male pheromone was placed beneath a chair in a dentist's waiting room, women tended to choose that chair to sit in but men avoided it. It also appears that a woman's ability to detect male pheromones naturally increases each month around the time of ovulation, when she's at her most fertile.

THINGS YOU DIDN'T KNOW ABOUT RELATIONSHIPS

○ You can't do anything about it now, but how close you were to your parents many years ago could be affecting your health decades later. Over 120 male Harvard students were asked how they felt about their parents. When their medical records were checked 35 years on, it was discovered that 87 per cent of the men who'd rated both their mothers and fathers negatively had gone on to develop a significant illness whereas only 25 per cent of men who'd rated both their parents positively had become ill. A similar study of students at the University of Arizona found positive perceptions of love and care from parents were associated with fewer psychiatric symptoms.

---

approach. For instance, if you're upset because you don't think your partner's earning enough money, you could say 'I'm worried about our financial situation and I feel very responsible for making sure we have enough money to get by. I'd feel a lot less stressed if you were able to increase your income.' (This approach is also probably better than saying something like 'Why don't you get a better job, you lazy slob?') Finally, it could be that your arguments reflect deeper problems with your relationship that you haven't yet tried to sort out. If this is the case, and you find it hard to address these issues, you could consider seeing a couples counselor.

I prefer my own company to that of other people
There's nothing inherently wrong with wanting to spend time on your own. Solitude can provide an opportunity to take part in many enjoyable and rewarding activities, such as listening to or playing music, painting, exercise, or simply watching your favorite videos. Being alone allows you to reflect on your life without interruption and to clarify what's currently going on. In fact, one characteristic of people with good mental health is that they tend to be comfortable being on their own; they don't need other people to distract them from their problems or to prop up a fragile sense of self-esteem. But since emotional well-being is generally also characterized by an ability to relate well to other people, you may want to think about whether your preference for solitude reflects how you really want to live your life or whether it's actually an attempt to make the best of a situation you're unhappy with deep-down.

CHAPTER 13

PILLOW TALK:
THE INS AND OUTS OF SEXUAL HEALTH

Imagine you've just had sex with a new partner, perhaps someone you met only recently. You've had your orgasm and you're lying in a strange bed, in the dark, staring quietly at the ceiling. What's going through your mind?

For a start, you're probably feeling pretty pleased with yourself. After all, to become sexually intimate so quickly must mean you're an attractive kind of guy. You relax as a wave of self-confidence passes through your body. Then you start to reflect on the sex itself. You wonder whether your partner was really having fun or if that orgasm was in reality more of a small hill than the mountain it seemed at the time. Then you remember how you listened out for the sounds of pleasure when you asked whether what you were doing felt nice. You also know that you enjoyed yourself, not least because you told your partner how you like your genitals to be touched and how you like to reach orgasm. You sense, too, that you both relaxed once you'd explained why you wanted to use a condom. As you pull the duvet up to your shoulders, you briefly recall how the two of you got the giggles at the moment of penetration and how you explained that sometimes, with a new partner, you can ejaculate more quickly than you'd like. (Although, once you'd said this, you felt it was a lot easier to delay your orgasm.) Your final thoughts before you drift into a peaceful sleep are about how you cuddled and chatted afterwards, shared a mug of tea, and agreed that it would be great to do this again soon.

Although there are many ways to have satisfying and fulfilling sex (what's just been described is only one of them), it remains an unusual experience for far too many of us. Fifty-six per cent of men are dissatisfied with their sex life and 83 per cent believe there's room for improvement in their sexual performance, according to a survey of 1500 men by a UK men's health magazine. Since enjoyable sex is so important to our sexual health, as well as our overall well-being, it's vital we find ways of improving our experiences between the sheets (or wherever else we choose to have them).

Why bother with sexual health?

○ You'll enjoy sex more. Developing a deeper understanding about what you want from sex, and becoming confident about asking for it, will almost certainly help you on your way to a more satisfying sex life.
○ You'll feel better about yourself. Once you stop measuring yourself against unrealistic objectives (a huge penis, earth-shattering orgasms, producing gallons of semen, etc.), you'll begin developing a greater sense of self-confidence about your body and what you can do with it.
○ You'll be less at risk of sexually transmitted infections (STIs) and other problems that can affect your sexual equipment such as erectile dysfunction (impotence) or premature ejaculation.
○ You could live longer. It's becoming increasingly clear that enjoying a fulfilled and intimate relationship can make an important contribution to good overall health and that a satisfying sex life can be a significant component of any such relationship. Effectively preventing, detecting, and treating diseases of your sexual and reproductive system could also help increase your lifespan.

What's going wrong?

Although modern men undoubtedly know far more about sex than their fathers, too many still have some rather strange ideas about it. Their heads are full of images from both mainstream movies and pornography that have convinced them that the key to a great sex life is simply to be constantly ready and eager and to have a massive, rock-hard penis, an encyclopaedic knowledge of every conceivable sexual position, as well as the ability to generate virtually endless amounts of thrusting. It's a process, moreover, that always culminates in penetration and a simultaneous multiple orgasm during which men ejaculate like hose-pipes; condoms aren't necessary because, somehow, women never get pregnant and nobody's at risk of catching an STI. It almost goes without saying that, in this version of good sex, men never have any doubts about their attractiveness, their ability to function sexually, or their sexual identity.

Attempting to model your sex life on what you see at the cinema, on video, or in magazines will almost certainly guarantee you bad sex. For a start, it's a fantasy: if we try to recreate this kind of sex in our own bedrooms we're setting ourselves up

REAL HEALTH FOR MEN

THE SCIENCE BIT

○ Sex helps keep you fit. Men's heart rates can rise rapidly during sex—from an average of 70–80 beats per minute at rest to 100–175 beats per minute during the build-up to orgasm and 110–180 beats during orgasm itself. The heart rates men experience during sex can be similar in intensity to those generated by vigorous aerobic exercise; in fact, an hour of passionate sex could easily burn off 360 calories, equivalent to about two pints of beer.

○ It helps you look younger. Couples who have sex at least three times a week look more than 10 years younger than couples who have sex twice a week, according to a 10-year study of over 3500 people aged 18–102 in Britain, Europe and the United States. After looking at all the factors that influence how old people look, sexual activity emerged as the most significant factor after physical and mental exercise.

○ Regular sex could keep you alive for longer. The more orgasms a man has, the longer he is likely to live, at least according to a study of over 900 middle-aged men in Wales. Men with a high frequency of orgasms during sexual intercourse (i.e. twice a week or more) are 50 per cent less likely to die from any cause within 10 years than men who have infrequent orgasms (less than one a month). Of course, these statistics could simply mean that healthy men have more sex—rather than it being the sex that keeps men healthy—but the figures are consistent with other research that strongly suggests that people with intimate relationships are healthier than those who feel lonely and isolated.

○ It boosts your hormones. Testosterone levels increase during and after sex, especially if there's a long period of foreplay. This not only helps maintain your sex drive but may also increase your fertility. Sex additionally boosts the levels of a little-known hormone known as DHEA (dehydroepiandrosterone). This is reputed to have a wide range of benefits, including improving your sense of physical and emotional well-being, increasing energy levels, and reducing the risk of heart problems.

for disappointment and failure. Secondly, the men who populate this make-believe world are there precisely because they aren't very much like most of us: they have muscular bodies, massive penises, know precisely how to satisfy any lover (even if they've only just met them), and can have sex for hours without ejaculating. If we try to measure ourselves against these latter-day Casanovas we'll probably end up with a case of severely dented self-confidence (as well as an extremely sore, over-used penis). And, finally, there's normally very little communication or intimacy between the partners we see on our screens. Their sex is cold and functional, and, although this kind of experience can sometimes feel right, most of us want much more from our sexual relationships.

The traditional male model of sex is also dangerous, both to ourselves and our partners. A lack of interest in, and knowledge of, STIs puts us all at increased risk of diseases like chlamydia, gonorrhea, and HIV (the virus that causes AIDS). Not sharing responsibility for contraception can expose women to the hazards and distress of an unplanned pregnancy (not to mention, potentially, years of motherhood) and men to the major responsibilities of fatherhood. What's more, if we don't understand how our sexual and reproductive system works, and what can go wrong with it, we're also much less likely to detect the early signs of a wide range of problems that can affect every part of our genitals (both inside and out).

My sex life's not sexy—how can I change?

BE MORE REALISTIC ABOUT SEX

This may mean jettisoning some of your cherished and long-held beliefs. For example:

- *Men should always be ready for sex.* Some men clearly have higher levels of sexual desire than others, but almost all men have a range of other needs in their lives (work, taking the children to school, sport, enjoying a drink) that are just as important to them as sex, if not more so. Stress, depression, and ill-health can also significantly reduce sex drive. In fact, loss of sexual desire is surprisingly common among men.
- *It's important to have a large penis.* Although many partners may get excited by the idea of a man with a larger penis, most are also perfectly satisfied by one of average length. Ninety per cent of women feel that penis size doesn't affect their orgasms, according to a survey conducted for a women's sex magazine.
- *Men's erections must be rock-hard.* Some may be but many aren't. About one in 10 men is consistently unable to achieve an erection hard enough for sex. Many more men will have occasional erection problems (perhaps as a result of stress or too much alcohol), while others will be able to get erections that are good enough for sex but certainly won't feel as if they're strong enough to support the roof of the Parthenon.

○ *Men should produce lots of semen.* They might in pornographic fiction, but in reality the average amount of fluid produced during ejaculation is about one teaspoonful (3 ml), although it can range from 1.5–6 ml. There's no obvious connection between how much you produce—or how far it shoots out—and your masculinity.

○ *Women can orgasm just from intercourse.* Just plugging your penis into a woman's vagina and wiggling it around may be enough to make some women orgasm but many will probably just lie there thinking about what they'd rather be watching on television. Even though most men have probably heard that women require clitoral stimulation in order to achieve an orgasm, they sometimes act as if they don't really believe it.

○ *All orgasms are stupendous.* Anyone who's honest will tell you this simply isn't true. Some orgasms are fantastic, others are barely noticeable, and they can vary from day to day almost as much as the weather. Men who are overweight and have sedentary jobs can find their orgasms become less powerful and pleasurable because of poor tone in their pelvic-floor muscles (these are responsible for expelling semen). 'Kegel' exercises are the best remedy: these simply involve regularly squeezing and relaxing the muscles you'd use to stop urinating in mid-stream.

FOCUS ON FUN AND PLEASURE, NOT PERFORMING

For many men, sex is like a climbing a mountain. You start at the base camp where you kiss and cuddle, and after a long slog up the lower slopes and then the steeper faces, you end up at the summit with penetration, ejaculation, and self-congratulation. Although it's certainly possible to have great sex this way, after a while it can easily become boring and predictable.

Key tips:
➲ Learn what you like. One good way of doing this is to spend more time masturbating. Seriously. By experimenting on your own you can discover much more about how you like to be touched. Once you've found out, tell your partner.
➲ Don't feel obliged to try different sexual positions. Most sex manuals are packed with examples of hundreds of different ways of having sex. Some of them will feel great, some will feel lousy, and some will be

A MAN'S GUIDE TO THE CLITORIS

Unless you've got a double-headed penis, it's difficult to have vaginal intercourse and stimulate the clitoris directly at the same time. That matters, because when it comes to a woman's orgasm, the clitoris is what really counts.

The visible part of the clitoris, located at the top of a woman's external genitals, is usually about the size of a small pea. But it's recently been discovered that the entire organ is very much larger. In fact, the visible 'glans' is connected to a hidden 'body' which is about as big as the first joint of the thumb. This body, in turn, has two 'arms,' each up to three-and-a-half inches long. Although the full role of the clitoris isn't yet understood, it's clear that it's at least as sensitive as the penis and just as significant during sex; indeed, both get bigger during sexual arousal. This shouldn't be surprising since both the clitoris and the penis are actually formed from the same tissues during our early days as a fetus.

Just as men's preferences for penile stimulation vary, so do women's preferences for their clitoris. Some find direct touching too sensitive while others like it to be rubbed or licked quite vigorously. No book can tell you how best to turn on a woman; you need to ask her to show or tell you. If she's willing to masturbate while you watch, this will give you very valuable clues.

unachievable by anyone who's not an Olympic gymnast. But the main problem with most information about sexual positions is that it reinforces the idea that sex is some kind of performance and that it's good only if you're constantly trying lots of different things. Variety can be important, but you should be guided primarily by what you and your partner find satisfying and exciting.

➲ Try not to rush toward intercourse. The word 'foreplay' is unfortunate since it strongly suggests that kissing, licking, sucking, and rubbing are somehow only preliminary stages in the run-up to the main event. Unless the goal of sex is pregnancy, there's no obvious or automatic reason why it should always include penetration. There are many other ways of having fun and achieving orgasm. It's often better simply to do what feels right, not what you think you should be doing after five, 10, or 15 minutes. It may be that you both want to spend 20 minutes just kissing or rubbing against each other with all your clothes on. Even if not doing what you've

---

TRY THESE ALTERNATIVES TO INTERCOURSE

○ Massage. Start by massaging your partner, tantalizingly leaving the genitals until last. Then let you partner massage you.

○ Mutual masturbation. Experiment, too, with a range of specially formulated lubricants. These now come in a bewilderingly large range of flavors and consistencies (including ones that replicate the body's sexual fluids); some even warm up as you use them.

○ Oral sex—an old favorite, but many men still see it as a starter rather than the main course.

○ Frotting—rubbing your bodies against each other.

○ Using sex toys—vibrators and dildos can get you both whirring. Try raiding your kitchen, too: cucumbers and bananas needn't be just for eating, and many people find ice cubes can excite their nipples and sexual organs.

All these options can be spiced up by dressing up, having sex in the bath or shower, trying different venues outside the home (e.g. in a car, in the countryside, in a hotel), role-playing, and just about anything else you can think of. You can try pretty much whatever you like providing your partner freely agrees.

---

always done feels artificial and a different kind of performance, stick with it. With time, this kind of sex should begin to feel more natural and spontaneous.

○ Try to relax and focus on the physical sensations of sex. That way, you're much more likely to enjoy sex—and give more pleasure to your partner. Try these suggestions:

○ Reduce your general levels of stress (see Chapter 10). It's generally not helpful to use sex as a distraction from whatever's worrying you; it won't tackle the underlying causes of your stress and it probably won't work anyway.

○ Regularly use simple relaxation techniques, such as deep breathing or tensing and relaxing your major muscle groups in turn.

○ Make sure that the sex you're having isn't adding to your stress levels. It probably isn't a good idea to end up in bed with someone you really don't like or who wants sex without a condom when you want to use one.

MASTURBATION: A USEFUL TOOL

It's certainly had a bad press. Victorian moralists believed masturbation was sinful 'self-abuse,' and doctors warned it could make you go blind or mad. Even in the 1990s, a US Surgeon General was forced out of office for suggesting that young people should learn about masturbation in school. Although few people now believe masturbation is wrong, many of us still feel slightly guilty about solo sex. Perhaps it's a legacy of the prudish past or maybe it's also because masturbation's seen as a sign of failure. After all, real men are supposed to have real sex, not make-believe sex with a bottle of oil and a box of tissues. But next time you feel inadequate about masturbating, remember that one survey of over 7000 men found that those having sex with a partner every day were *more* likely to masturbate once a week or more than men who rarely or never had sex with a partner.

Masturbation can be fun and relaxing—crucially, there's no pressure to perform—and it's also completely safe (unless you happen to be turned on by cheese graters).

Key tips:
- Make sure you have some uninterrupted private time. It's difficult to enjoy masturbating if you're expecting an important telephone call or your parents are about to visit.
- Have a relaxing bath or shower. Dry yourself but don't get dressed.
- Lie down on your bed. Make sure the room's comfortably warm; you may want to create a more sensual atmosphere by drawing the curtains, lighting some candles, playing background music, and locking out the cat.
- Using some moisturizing lotion or massage oil, start to massage gently your face, hands, arms, legs, and feet. Then massage your stomach and chest. You don't need to be thinking about anything sexy at this stage; try to focus on relaxing and the physical sensations of the massage instead.
- When you feel ready, start to massage your nipples, then your scrotum, perineum (the area between your scrotum and anus), and penis. It's fine if sexual thoughts enter your mind, but don't try and force them.
- Try not to focus only on your penis. Go back over other parts of your body, noticing which areas you especially enjoy touching.

MASTURBATION: A USEFUL TOOL

⤴ Experiment with touching your penis in different ways—varying the speed, pressure, and direction—again noticing what feels particularly good. Try to touch all of your penis, not just the head or shaft.

⤴ You don't have to produce an erection and you don't have to go all the way to orgasm, unless you want to. If you decide to ejaculate, just before you do so, stop masturbating for a couple of minutes until the feeling subsides before starting again. See if this creates any heightened sensations.

⤴ Notice how you like to touch yourself immediately before and during your orgasm. This is particularly important information that you could pass on to a partner.

At first, you may find this exercise difficult, or even a bit silly. If so, don't give up, but try it again in a few days. Make a mental note of what you enjoyed: it could improve the quality of your masturbation as well as sex with a partner.

○ Don't use mind-games to try to stop yourself ejaculating too quickly. They reduce your enjoyment of sex—let's face it, thinking about your dream soccer team or quadratic equations might be interesting activities but they aren't exactly erotic (at least, not for most of us)—and there are much better ways of tackling premature ejaculation (see page 251).

○ Focus on the 'here-and-now' when you're masturbating or having sex. Although there's nothing wrong with sexual fantasy, try having sex without it for a while (and dump any pornography, too). This could help you become more aware of the physical sensations you experience during sex and relax better into them.

○ Don't hold back from moving around as much as you need to when you're having sex (yes, men are allowed to squirm with pleasure) or moaning and groaning.

○ Try not to take sex too seriously. We often approach it as if we were about to race a Grand Prix or attend a religious service. Although sex is a supremely important activity, it can also be absurd and funny. Having a laugh during and after sex—so long as it's not at your or your partner's expense—can help you feel relaxed as well as much more in touch with what's going on.

COMMUNICATE WITH YOUR PARTNER

Whether you've just started a sexual relationship or have been in one for 30 years, it's still important to talk about it. You'd probably discuss what color to paint your living room, what car to buy, or where to go on holiday, so why not talk to your partner about sex, too?

Key tips:
- ➲ Find ways of communicating better with your partner about every aspect of your relationship (see Chapter 12). This should also help to improve your sex life.
- ➲ Express how much you like your partner's body. You don't only have to do this in bed. Putting an arm round your partner's shoulder, squeezing their hand or initiating a kiss are all important. Explain why you find them desirable and sexy, perhaps not just in terms of the obvious features but also the things that appeal specifically to you (e.g. the curve of their lip, that mole on the inner thigh, the way they walk). If your partner does the same to you, make sure you acknowledge it rather than seem to take it for granted.
- ➲ Develop a physically intimate relationship that extends beyond sex. If a couple are relaxed with, and enjoy, each other's bodies in non-sexual ways, this can have significant sexual benefits. Simply holding hands or cuddling while watching television can create a greater sense of intimacy, as can learning how to provide a simple but relaxing massage.
- ➲ Talk about what you want in bed. This is best done without criticism or blame, so don't say something like 'I hate the way you never suck my prick.' You're much more likely to get a positive response if you say something like 'Seeing your lips round my cock drives me wild.' If your partner really doesn't feel comfortable about oral sex, you could try suggesting some sort of compromise (e.g. your partner licks the inside of your thighs while masturbating you).
- ➲ Be aware of what your partner wants, rather than make assumptions. One way is simply to say 'Does that feel good?'; another is to do more of whatever produces pleasurable noises ('mmmm' or 'ahhhhh') and less of whatever produces silence or 'ugh' sounds. Watch out for physical signs, too: if your partner's nipples stiffen or genitals moisten, then you're probably doing okay; however, you should try something different if you feel your hand, head, or penis being pushed away. Ask what your partner wants, too—and take it seriously. You can't really expect your partner to do what you'd like if you're not prepared to reciprocate (or at least discuss it).

➲ Share your sexual fantasies. You may need to be sensitive about this—your partner might not appreciate it if all your fantasies are about a previous lover, for instance, or involve herds of wild animals—but sharing can be both a sign of trust and a clear signal of your sexual desires. But you can't expect your partner automatically to agree to act out all your fantasies (or vice versa). Not everyone likes being covered in strawberries and cream. Again, it's something to discuss and reach an agreement about.

➲ Discuss how often you and your partner want sex. Often, at the start of a relationship, a couple will have sex at almost every opportunity. After a few months, however, sex may steadily become less frequent. This is a normal development but it can be a time when differences emerge in partners' levels of sexual desire. This can cause frustration and resentment in the partner who feels deprived, and guilt and anger in the partner who feels pressured to have sex when not feeling aroused. Many couples in this position find it helpful to agree a mutually acceptable arrangement. It's also important to remember that this needn't exclude non-sexual physical intimacy at other times.

➲ If you find it hard to talk about your sexual needs with a partner, perhaps because you feel embarrassed or ashamed, you could start by trying to have a more abstract conversation about sex. If you see an article in a newspaper or a television program that deals with sexual issues, you might discuss what you think of it. Over time, as you become more at ease with talking about sex, you may feel ready to take the risk of being more personal.

➲ If it feels impossible to discuss sex at all then it's more than likely that your sex life is not all it could be and that it won't improve much over time. But you don't have to give up. Perhaps the best way of breaking through the barrier is for you and your partner to see a couples counselor or a sex therapist. Don't worry: you won't end up being forced to have sex on his or her office floor, but you should find it'll become much easier to explore, and sort out, your sexual inhibitions.

➲ However, and whatever, you communicate, one thing is clear: it's vital to be honest. Pretending you're happy with your sex life when you're not can easily begin to cause resentment and even anger; it can end up putting a strain on the entire relationship. Honesty's especially important if you have a sexual problem, such as erectile dysfunction (impotence). However uncomfortable it feels to be honest, it's more than likely that the long-term consequences of dishonesty will feel much, much worse.

BE RESPONSIBLE

Your sex life will be a lot happier and healthier if you take good care of yourself—and those you have sex with.

Key tips:
- ➲ Wise up. There are many health problems which can affect the sexual and reproductive organs. At least one man in three will have some sort of prostate-gland disorder during his lifetime, about the same proportion will experience a sexual dysfunction, and one in 20 will be affected by fertility problems (such as a low sperm count). Each year, one in 100 men is likely to catch an STI such as gonorrhea, chlamydia, or HIV. Although testicular cancer affects just one in 450 men, its incidence has doubled in the last 20 years and looks set to

BED BUGS – The main sexually transmitted infections (STIs)

Chlamydia

Symptoms	Often unnoticed, but can include discharge from penis and pain when urinating. The eyes can swell up if infected.
Cause	Bacterial infection.
Prevention	Use a condom.
Treatment	Antibiotic.
Outlook	Good, although the infection can spread to the testicles and prostate gland. There are also long-term risks to partners: chlamydia can cause infertility in women.

Gonorrhea

Symptoms	Often none, although typically there's a white/yellow discharge from the penis and pain when urinating. Oral infection can cause a sore throat. It's also possible to develop rectal gonorrhea.
Cause	Bacterial infection.
Prevention	Use a condom.
Treatment	Antibiotic.
Outlook	Good, although the infection can spread to the testicles and prostate gland.

BED BUGS – The main sexually transmitted infections (STIs)

Herpes

Symptoms	Blisters around the mouth, penis, or anus. These burst, then a scab forms and heals within 10–14 days. The blisters may recur. There may also be flu-like aches and pains, particularly when the blisters first appear.
Cause	A virus.
Prevention	Avoid sex with anyone who has a cold sore or blisters. Using a condom should help if you do have sex.
Treatment	The virus can't be eradicated but your immune system will normally keep it suppressed. Special tablets and creams can make the blisters go away more quickly. Avoid stress and sunbathing—these can trigger an attack.
Outlook	A depressing condition, but one that can, with care, be kept under control.

Hepatitis A

Symptoms	Six weeks after infection you may experience mild flu-like symptoms. You may also have a fever or diarrhea, your urine may go dark, and your faeces turn pale. Your skin and eyes can become yellow.
Cause	A virus found in excrement.
Prevention	Have a vaccination. Otherwise, avoid any type of sex that might bring your skin into contact with faeces.
Treatment	Plenty of rest, a nourishing diet, and no alcohol.
Outlook	It can make you very ill, but most people recover after a long convalescence.

Hepatitis B

Symptoms	A flu-like illness, no appetite, pain in the abdomen, your urine may go dark, and your faeces turn pale. Your skin and eyes can become yellow.
Cause	A virus transmitted through vaginal, anal, and oral sex as well as kissing.

BED BUGS – The main sexually transmitted infections (STIs)

Prevention   Have a vaccination. Condoms will help reduce the risk.

Treatment   Plenty of rest, a nourishing diet, and no alcohol.

Outlook   It can make you very ill, but most people recover after a long convalescence.

HIV

Symptoms   There are no symptoms immediately after infection, but there may be a flu-like illness a few weeks later. There may be no further symptoms for several years, although it's likely that diseases and infections will start to appear as the immune system weakens.

Cause   A virus that weakens the immune system. It's transmitted sexually through semen, vaginal fluid, and blood.

Prevention   Use a condom during penetrative intercourse. Avoid oral sex if you have sores in your mouth or throat. (See page 191–2 for more information on safer sex.) A vaccine could be available within 10 years.

Treatment   There's no cure, but drugs can lower the amount of the virus in the body (although these don't work for everybody). Many of the illnesses associated with HIV can be treated or kept under control.

Outlook   Good in the short and medium term; uncertain in the longer term. But new and more effective drugs are constantly becoming available.

Non-specific urethritis

Symptoms   Often none, but sometimes a white discharge from the penis or pain when urinating.

Cause   Bacteria—the exact type isn't known (which is why the condition is called 'non-specific').

Prevention   Use a condom.

Treatment   Antibiotics.

Outlook   Good.

BED BUGS – The main sexually transmitted infections (STIs)

Pubic lice

Symptoms	'Crabs' cause itching around pubic hair and sometimes a rash. (They can spread to other areas of body hair, but not the head.)
Cause	Small insects that feed on human blood. They're no bigger than a pin-head when fully grown.
Prevention	None, unless you avoid touching your partner's genitals.
Treatment	Special insecticidal lotion.
Outlook	Good.

Syphilis

Symptoms	Although it doesn't always produce symptoms, the typical pattern is: first, a painless red sore on the penis, testicles, mouth, throat, or anus; this disappears after 3–6 weeks. The second-phase symptoms include a skin rash, fever, headaches, and hair loss. These symptoms can come and go for up to two years. In the final stage, often years later, the disease damages the nervous system, heart, and brain.
Cause	A bacteria that lives in warm, moist areas like the urethra (the tube running through the penis) and the bowel.
Prevention	Use a condom.
Treatment	Antibiotics.
Outlook	Good, if treated early. Any damage caused during the later stages of the disease is permanent.

Warts

Symptoms	Small growths, either singly or in groups, on the penis and/or around the anus. As they grow, they become cauliflower shaped.
Cause	Viruses that live in the skin (known as the human papillomaviruses, or HPVs).
Prevention	Use a condom.
Treatment	Freezing with liquid nitrogen, using a special anti-viral 'paint' or cream, surgical or laser removal.

BED BUGS – The main sexually transmitted infections (STIs)

Outlook   The warts can be removed, but the virus lives on in the body and the problem can recur. Warts also create a risk of cervical cancer in women and anal cancer in men who receive anal intercourse.

The symptoms of many STIs aren't always obvious, can take a long time to show up, or can appear briefly and then disappear. If you're sexually active with more than one person, or you're about to have sex with a new partner, you should seriously consider having a routine STI check-up. If you think you have an STI, you must see a doctor: it's difficult for you to diagnose your condition accurately, and in any event it's impossible for it to be effectively treated without drugs available only on prescription.

continue to rise. One survey found that just over half of men knew that prostate cancer was a disease that could only affect men; under one-third of men knew even one of the major symptoms. The more you know about these problems, the easier it will be for you to prevent them arising in the first place and to detect and treat them if they do.

The symptoms of the main STIs are described on the preceding pages. Whether or not you're sexually active, you should also look out for symptoms of other important sexual health problems. These include:

- ○ Lumps, scars, or bending in the penis.
- ○ A discharge from the penis.
- ○ A tight foreskin.
- ○ The inability to achieve an erection.
- ○ Painful erections or an erection that won't go down.
- ○ Rapid or delayed ejaculation during sex.
- ○ Loss of sexual desire.
- ○ Problems with urination: pain, increased frequency, a weak urinary stream, or blood in the urine.
- ○ Pain during ejaculation.
- ○ Blood in the semen.
- ○ Testicular pain or lumps or a change in size, shape, or firmness of one or both testicles.
- ○ Sores, blisters, ulcers, or growths on the genitals.

Chapter 16 contains more information about these symptoms and what they could mean. But if you have an erection that won't go down (priapism), or acute pain in the testicles (this could be a testicular torsion), see a doctor as soon as possible.

○ Have 'safer sex', unless you're sure both you and your partner are HIV negative (i.e. not infected with the virus). Essentially this is a way of behaving sexually that minimizes the risks of transmitting the virus. As discussed, earlier, it's called 'safer' rather than 'safe' sex as it involves greatly reducing the risk rather than eliminating it completely. Safer sex will also reduce your chances of contracting or passing on many other STIs.

○ Be assertive. Choosing safer sex can be difficult. Even if you want to use a condom, you might feel embarrassed if you're not confident you know how to put one on; alternatively, you might be worried about losing your erection. (See page 194 for tips on using a condom.) On the other hand, your partner might not want to have sex with a condom. You might then think that if you insist on using one, it implies that you've got an infection or that you don't trust your partner. It can all get very complicated and there's no easy way to talk about this. But if your partner's reluctant to use a condom, the only viable strategy is for you to say you're not prepared to have penetrative sex without one.

○ Be open. If you have an STI, it's your responsibility to tell your partner(s). They can then decide if they want to have sex with you and, if so, how. If they've already had sex with you, they may need to get themselves checked to see if they've been infected. You might think that it's not up to you to tell partners on the grounds that it's their responsibility to make sure that whatever they do is safe. You could also be worried that nobody will want to have sex with you if they know you have an STI or that they will be angry with you if you tell them they've been exposed to a risk of infection. Perhaps your best guide is to ask yourself if you'd want a partner to tell you of any potential risk to your health and to act accordingly.

○ Be fully involved in decisions about contraception. Too many men still see contraception as a woman's rather than a couple's issue. Almost two-thirds believe women are 'mainly' responsible for contraception according to UK Health Education Authority research. A lack of interest in contraception not only annoys women (quite understandably) but can also mean that a couple ends up using a form of contraception that doesn't meet both of their needs when it comes to preventing pregnancy, minimizing the risks of STIs, or, importantly, simply having fun. Given that about a dozen methods of birth control are now widely available, it should be possible to find at least one that feels right.

Sexual activity	Risk of HIV transmission	You need to know
Fingering	Low	Avoid if you have cuts or sores on the finger that's in your partner's vagina or anus.
Food	Low	Take care if you're sharing a cucumber or banana as a sex toy (see below). The main risk of eating ice cream off your partner's genitals is that you'll put on weight.
Frottage (body rubbing)	Low	Don't let sexual fluids come finto contact with any cuts or sores.
Kissing (mouth to mouth)	Low	Saliva's no risk so it doesn't matter how far your tongue goes down your partner's throat (but be careful of any bleeding around the mouth).
Lovebites	Low	But don't chomp so hard you break the skin—you can't transmit HIV from saliva but the wound might come into contact with infected vaginal juices, semen, or blood.
Massage	None	Remember that oils can rot latex condoms.
Masturbation (solo)	None	It's as safe as it gets.

Sexual activity	Risk of HIV transmission	You need to know
Oral sex	Low (in general)	Avoid it if there are any cuts, sores, bleeding gums or ulcers in or around the mouth, or throat infections. Cunnilingus should be avoided if a woman is menstruating.
Phone sex	None	The only risk is being ripped off by a commercial service.
Rimming (licking your partner's anus)	Low	But not a good idea without some sort of barrier (e.g. a cut-open condom) since it can expose you to other viruses, bacteria, and parasites.
Sex toys (e.g. dildos)	Low	Clean them thoroughly before they're shared (or put condoms on them—it can be easier to change the condom than take the toy to the bathroom).
Unprotected penetrative sex (anal or vaginal)	High	This is the main way in which HIV is transmitted. The best method of reducing the risk is always to wear a condom.
Watersports (playing with urine)	Low	Urine is generally a sterile fluid and contains at most minute quantities of HIV.

○ Consider a vasectomy, especially if you're sure you've completed your family (or that you don't want to start one). It's an extremely effective form of contraception—the long-term failure rate is just 1 in 3000—and you'll notice no difference in the volume, color, or consistency of your semen and no change in sex drive or the experience of ejaculation and orgasm. On the downside, however, a vasectomy must be considered irreversible: although many men do have successful (and expensive) reversal operations, there are no guarantees that normal fertility will return. There may also be bruising, swelling, and infection after a vasectomy, and as many as one in 10 men may suffer from long-term scrotal pain. The procedure normally involves a local anesthetic to numb the area followed by a small cut in the skin in the middle or on both sides of the scrotum. The vas deferens—the tubes leading from the testicles to the penis—are then pulled through the incision, cut, and the ends securely tied to prevent sperm becoming part of the seminal fluid. It takes time to work: you'll have sperm tests at 12 and 16 weeks after the snip, and if there are still live sperm in your semen, you must produce samples every four weeks until two consecutive tests give the all clear.

DEVELOP GREATER SELF-CONFIDENCE ABOUT YOUR SEXUALITY

The better you feel about yourself, the more you're likely to enjoy sex. You'll probably feel less inhibited, more open to new ideas and experiences, and better able to tell your partner what you want during sex.

Key tips:
➲ Feel good about what you've got. If you believe you need to look or behave like Keanu Reeves to enjoy sex then you're setting yourself up for an inferiority complex that's larger than Rambo's biceps. The vast majority of men aren't like Keanu, just as most women don't look very much like Catherine Zeta Jones or Naomi Campbell. It might seem a bit of a cliché, but your attractiveness is more related to your personality than your physical appearance. If you feel attractive, you'll probably look attractive to others. (See Chapter 15.)
➲ Be honest about your sexuality. While scientists struggle to understand the roots of our sexual identity—it's still not clear whether we're straight, gay, or bisexual because of our genetic make-up, for instance, or as a result of our experiences as we grow up—it's beyond doubt that human males exhibit a very diverse range of sexual preferences. Most men are attracted to women

HOW TO USE A CONDOM

There's much more to using a condom than simply tearing open the packet and sticking it on your penis. If you're new to condoms, practice when you're home alone.

Key tips:
- Shop around. Condoms come in different sizes, shapes, thicknesses, and flavors. Experiment to see which are best for you. If you're having anal sex, always go for a thicker condom.
- Check the use-by date as condoms can deteriorate with age.
- Make sure the condom meets recognized safety requirements (the British Standard Kitemark symbol on condoms manufactured in the UK is generally acknowledged to be the highest standard in the world). Never trust condoms that are shaped like animals, are luminous in the dark, or play tunes when you take them out of the packet. These are novelty products, recommended only for blowing up, sticking over your head, or making water bombs.
- Open the packet carefully, even if you're excited. Although condoms are very strong, they can be torn by fingernails, rings, or even rough skin.
- Wait until your penis is fully erect before you put on the condom.
- Because seminal fluid can come out of your penis before you ejaculate, you should put the condom on before you attempt penetration.
- Make sure you put it on the right way round. The best method is to hold the closed end between the thumb and forefinger of one hand and squeeze the air out. Then, using the other hand, place the condom on the tip of your penis and unroll it fully down the shaft.
- Slap on plenty of water-based lubricant for extra pleasure. Don't use petroleum jelly or massage oil—they can rot latex remarkably quickly. (Although, confusingly, you can safely use oil-based lubes with polyurethane condoms.)
- Check it regularly. In some sexual positions, the condom can roll up so make sure it's still in position during sex.
- Remove it carefully. Because your penis goes limp soon after you've ejaculated, you should hold the base of the condom firmly in place and withdraw before any semen can leak out of the condom. It's not compulsory to show your partner how much you've produced; in fact, it's probably better to wrap the condom in a tissue and throw it away in a bin. (Don't chuck it down the toilet—used condoms are a nightmare for sewage companies and can end up on beaches.)

SHOULD YOU HAVE AN HIV TEST?

If you're worried that you could be HIV positive (i.e. you have been infected with HIV), a blood test will tell you one way or the other. If you discover that you are HIV positive, you can then get medical advice and treatment that could make a big difference to your health. You'll also be able to take steps to protect anyone you have sex with and inform any past sexual partners who might have been at risk. If you find you are HIV negative, however, and you're sure that your partner is too, then you can safely ditch the condoms and start having unprotected sex—unless, of course, you're using them as a form of contraception. (But you must remember that it takes three months for HIV to become detectable in a blood test, so if you've been infected in that period the test could show incorrectly that you're HIV negative.)

One big argument against having a test is that it can be a very frightening experience, whatever the result. (If you do go ahead, you may want to consider getting the support of a close friend as well as making sure you have the test at a clinic that offers counseling before and after the result. Many clinics also offer a same-day results service, which some people find helps reduce the stress of waiting.) You'll need to be confident you can cope if you do get bad news; you might want to wait if you're suffering from other sources of stress at the moment. If you are HIV positive, it could well affect your relationships with your partner and anyone else you choose to tell. Some employers may also be reluctant to offer you a job, you could find it harder to obtain insurance, and a few countries place restrictions on the entry of people known to be HIV positive.

It can be a difficult decision, and there's no right or wrong course of action. Only you can decide, but you might find it helpful to get more information and advice from an organization specializing in HIV issues.

only, but a significant minority is sexually interested only in other men, while a third group is attracted to both men and women. None of these preferences is better, more moral, or healthier than any other; what's most important is that a man should feel comfortable with his sexual preference.

Many straight men worry that enjoying sexual stimulation of their nipples, anus or prostate gland means that they must somehow be gay, even though they're attracted only to women. The reality is that all men—straight, gay, and bisexual—have many erogenous zones besides their penis. The fact that more gay men than straight men enjoy stimulation of their prostate means only that straight men tend to have a much more limited view of what's acceptable and unacceptable between the sheets. In fact, there are many ways in which a heterosexual man can enjoy prostate stimulation besides having another man's penis inserted into his rectum (a partner's finger or a dildo will do perfectly well).

A more distressing problem affects men who know they're gay but can't admit it to their friends, relatives, or sometimes even to themselves. In some cases, these men may live with women, and perhaps have children too, and appear to the world to be happily heterosexual. Their difficulty in 'coming out' may be linked to feelings of guilt, shame, or a fear of hurting, or being rejected by, others. It could also be related to the fact that, despite the moves toward greater equality for homosexuals in most Western countries in the past 30 years, gay men and lesbians are still widely subjected to discrimination, prejudice, and even violence. For many gay and bisexual men, coming out remains a stressful and dangerous step.

Men who are unsure of their sexual orientation, or who feel hesitant about coming out, can contact a wide variety of organizations for advice and support. Although it's difficult to generalize, it does seem as if most men ultimately benefit from being more open about their sexuality. The stress of living a lie about such a fundamental part of one's life cannot be over-estimated.

What's stopping you?

I find foreplay boring

Although it can be great to have fast sex occasionally, if you keep skipping foreplay your partner might well soon start skipping you. There could be four explanations for your feelings about foreplay. The first is that you still believe in the outdated male notion that foreplay is largely an irrelevance and that what really counts is simply sticking your penis in. Secondly, you may never have tried foreplay and therefore could remain unaware of its many pleasures. Thirdly, you may never have learned that you have many erogenous zones besides your penis (e.g. your nipples, testicles, thighs, anus, lips, buttocks, and abdomen). Finally, it's possible that you're scheduling sex as if it's a meeting and not leaving yourself enough time to get into it. Whatever the reason, take a chance—try foreplay and see what you've been missing.

Condoms ruin sex
Most men find that sex with a condom doesn't feel the same as sex without one; there is, inevitably, some effect on sensation. However, wearing a condom gives you one big advantage: you do know that the sex you're having is much, much safer. You can also try and spice up your condom experience by asking your partner to put it on for you—you can even make this part of sex play (e.g. a shared sexual fantasy) rather than something that can often seem like a medical procedure. Adding lubrication can also help improve sensitivity. Some men claim that because condoms help delay ejaculation they actually lead to a more powerful orgasm.

I feel very inhibited around sex
It's common occasionally to feel embarrassed or shy, but if your feelings are stronger and getting in the way of sex then you need to find out why. Some men who had very religious or prudish parents have been brought up to believe that sex is somehow shameful or dirty. Others may have been punished if caught playing with their penis as a child or masturbating when a teenager, leaving them with the belief that sex is wrong. A bad first sexual experience, such as being criticized by a partner for coming too quickly or not being able to get an erection, could also cause problems, as could a history of sexual abuse. The best way to deal with sexual inhibitions is to see a sex therapist or counselor.

I'm worried I've picked up a dose of the clap but I'm scared about the tests a clinic will want to carry out
You'll probably be offered a range of tests to check for all the major STIs. Gonorrhea and chlamydia are usually checked by a swab pushed into the tip of the urethra (the tube running through your penis). There's no denying it stings—and rather more than cheap after-shave—but it doesn't last more than a few seconds. (And despite what some blokes say, the swab certainly isn't the size of a coat hanger.) But if the idea of this really bothers you, ask if the clinic can use a more recently introduced urine test for these diseases. Other diseases, such as syphilis and HIV, require a blood test. If you're needle-phobic, make sure you tell the doctor or nurse so they can be as gentle and reassuring as possible. However scared you are by the tests, you should remember it's likely that you'll be even more worried by the idea of having an infection that remains undiagnosed and untreated.

THINGS YOU DIDN'T KNOW ABOUT SEXUAL HEALTH

○ Men have more sex around Christmas, with another peak during the summer vacations, according to a study of abortions, condom sales, and the diagnosis of STIs.

○ Men with larger organs might not be boasting when they say their condoms are too tight—sheaths do vary considerably in size and shape (as well as thickness) and research suggests men do find some much more comfortable than others. A UK study that looked at 200 men's experiences of using four different condoms found the smallest-diameter condom was least popular (although those who found it fitted were still enthusiastic about it), while similar proportions of men had a clear preference for contoured, flared, or straight-sided condoms. If you find one type of condom uncomfortable, shop around until you find another that suits you better. Widely available condoms vary in length from 168–191 mm while circumferences range from 98–111 mm.

○ Men with the least symmetrical hands—where one hand isn't the mirror image of the other—have the lowest sperm counts and the poorest levels of sperm movement, according to a study by scientists at Liverpool University in the UK. Men who produced virtually no sperm had asymmetries of up to four millimeters between their hands. The same research also found that men whose ring fingers are much longer than their index fingers tend to have higher levels of testosterone. As yet, there's no convincing explanation for these findings.

○ The number and quality of sperm is highest between 5 and 7pm, according to an Italian fertility clinic. This happily coincides with the time women are most likely to ovulate (between 3 and 7pm). More than 75 per cent of the men tested at the clinic had sperm concentrations that were 35 per cent higher in the late afternoon.

CHAPTER 14

INJURY TIME:

THE ILL MAN'S GUIDE
TO THRIVING AND SURVIVING

ew westerns or war films are complete without a scene in which the badly wounded hero dismisses his injuries as a mere 'flesh wound' and carries on to rescue the innocent and defeat the enemy. Medical attention is sought only when the mission is complete, and recovery is usually miraculously fast. As soon as he can stand, our hero is pestering his doctor to be allowed to saddle up or return to the front-line. He suffers no lasting physical effects, and his mind remains untraumatized by the whole experience. Within a few days it's as if the whole thing never happened. Clearly, real men don't let a little (or even a big) health problem stop them getting the job done.

But this scenario bears as little resemblance to reality as a painting by Picasso. However much we might like to pretend otherwise, real-life health problems—and their treatments—can be inconvenient, uncomfortable, painful, worrying, disabling, and unpredictable. Whether you've got the flu or cancer, there are no 'magic bullet' treatments that can quickly get you back on your feet. Recovery is often a slow process: it's not for nothing that people with health problems are called 'patients.' But there are also many ways in which we can improve the way we cope with ill-health. The experience of illness can be about far more than simply feeling sorry for ourselves and passively waiting for the first signs of healing. If we can fully accept that we have a health problem, and focus on how best to tackle whatever's wrong with us, then we're much more likely to get better—and faster.

Am I really ill?

Before you can start recovering from an illness, you first need to acknowledge that you could actually be ill. This can sometimes be difficult because, if you normally feel reasonably healthy, you might well tend to dismiss any symptoms as trivial or irrelevant. Regular headaches can easily be attributed to stress or long hours at the computer and constant fatigue explained away as the result of too many late nights. And, of course, these are all plausible explanations. They are also explanations that, if you are in fact ill, could delay your treatment and leave you with even greater health problems.

Key tips:
- ➲ Acknowledge your vulnerability. Yes, it can happen to you too. However much you might want to believe otherwise, you will almost inevitably get ill at some point. Remember that even Superman, the Man of Steel, can expire if he's exposed to rocks of green kryptonite.
- ➲ Be honest. Embarrassment and fear about being ill can make men deny their symptoms, both to themselves and other people, even though they know deep-down that there might be a serious problem. Sometimes the truly courageous course of action is to be open and up front about what's going on rather than trying to hide it and carry on regardless.
- ➲ Get information. If you're worried, read up on your symptoms. Most bookstores and libraries stock medical books aimed at the general public. Take a look at reputable Internet websites: these are now an invaluable (and huge) additional source of information. See Chapter 16 of this book for information on a range of men's health problems.
- ➲ Talk to other people. Ask a partner, relatives, friends, or colleagues what they think about your symptoms. Try calling confidential telephone helplines that deal with health problems. Other perspectives can be useful in helping you think more clearly what might be going on and what you should do.
- ➲ Remember Rudolph Valentino. The 1920s heart-throb died in his early 30s after refusing medical help for far too long. He was in his hotel room when he suddenly felt an intense stabbing pain in his side. He spent the night in agony but saw a doctor only when his temperature soared and he became semi-delirious. By then, he had a perforated stomach ulcer, a ruptured appendix, and a serious infection that had already spread throughout the lining of the abdominal wall. He survived for only eight days.

Should I see a doctor?

If you're in any doubt about whether your condition could be serious, or if you're in pain, get medical advice. Ignore any worries that you'll be wasting the doctor's time or that he or she will think you're a hypochondriac—neither is likely to be true. But if you feel you need an excuse to see a doctor, book yourself a routine check-up and you can then raise your particular worry between the blood pressure and cholesterol tests.

Remember one obvious fact: the earlier almost any illness is detected and treated, the greater your chances of recovery. This is especially true in the case of a heart attack: one study found that patients treated in the first hour after the symptoms start are seven times less likely to die than if treated later. But other research, looking at over 2400 heart attack patients, found that 40 per cent waited more than six hours before going to a hospital.

Some men have particular concerns about seeing a doctor if they have problems with their genitals. Apart from the embarrassment most of us feel about taking our clothes off in front of a stranger, they also worry about the possibility that they might have some sort of sexual response (i.e. an erection). This is extremely unlikely for one obvious physiological reason: even if your doctor is gorgeous, your feelings of stress or anxiety will interrupt the messages the brain sends to your penis in order to make an erection possible.

Is it serious?

Most of the illnesses you'll suffer from will be minor and only temporarily inconvenient. Most colds and stomach upsets will clear up within a week, for instance, and you can expect to be fully recovered from a bout of flu within a fortnight. Discovering you have a rather more serious health problem is never a pleasant experience, although sometimes receiving a clear diagnosis can feel like something of a relief if you've had unpleasant symptoms without a clear idea of what was causing them. Your feelings about a diagnosis will probably depend on exactly what's wrong with you and how serious it is. These are some of the questions you may want to ask your doctor:

- ○ Is the diagnosis definite? Is there any chance it could be wrong? What's the evidence for it?
- ○ Exactly what is this problem?
- ○ Is it serious? How will it affect me? Can it get worse—and by how much?
- ○ If there's any pain, can it be controlled?

GETTING THE BEST FROM YOUR DOC

Because doctors are busy people, you need to know how to make the most of the time you're with them. It might help if you think about your consultations as you would about a meeting at work—a bit of forward planning can make a huge difference to the outcome.

Key tips:

➲ Make a mental (or written) note of all your symptoms before you meet the doctor. Leave nothing out, however trivial or embarrassing it might seem.

➲ If you've got several worries, talk about the most significant first. Don't leave mentioning the massive ulcer on your penis until you're backing out of the door.

➲ Don't try and use medical jargon you don't fully understand to impress the doctor. If he or she uses terms that baffle you, ask for an explanation. Requesting more information doesn't mean you're an idiot.

➲ If you're worried that you might have a particular illness, ask.

➲ If your doctor suggests further tests, find out what they're for and what they will entail.

➲ If you're given a prescription, make sure you know how to take the drug and what any side-effects might be. Make sure you know when and how often to take it and whether you may need to lay off alcohol. If you're unhappy about what's proposed, ask about any alternatives.

➲ If your doctor suggests referring you to a specialist, make sure you know why and ask how long you're likely to have to wait for an appointment.

➲ Before you leave, make sure you have had full answers. If you feel the doctor has give you a very vague diagnosis—'back trouble', for example, or 'a sensitive stomach'—ask for more details. After all, you wouldn't be very happy if a builder told you simply that your house had 'roof problems'.

➲ If you're dissatisfied with your doctor's advice, you can always ask for a second opinion.

➲ If you're consistently unhappy with your doctor—perhaps because the consultations always seemed too rushed or you feel as if you're being patronized—find a new one.

➲ See you doctor as a colleague rather than a boss. Don't just accept whatever he or she says, but ask questions, challenge (politely) what you disagree with, and make your own choices about the treatment you want. It's your body and you can decide what will—or won't—be done to it.

○ What are the treatments? Do I have any choices? What's the evidence of their effectiveness and do they have any side-effects? How long do the treatments take?
○ Where can I be treated? Where am I likely to receive the best treatment?
○ What are my chances of being cured?

You may not think of all the questions you need to ask at the time you receive your diagnosis, but you can raise them at the next meeting with the doctor who's treating you.

Dealing with bad news

If you've just been told you've got a serious or potentially life-threatening condition, the chances are you'll be in a state of shock. Your mind might go numb and you could well find it hard to believe what you've just been told. This is an entirely normal response to frightening news.

Once you've begun to acknowledge that you have a problem, you may go on to feel very alone and isolated. You might feel distant from your partner, friends, and family. You also could experience feelings of shame, guilt, anger, fear, and depression. It can take some time before you're able to come to terms with your illness, accept how it might change your life, and begin to think more constructively or positively about it.

Key tips:
➲ Accept that it's okay to feel scared. Only a robot could remain unfazed at the news that its circuits are malfunctioning. Don't get trapped into trying to repress your fear—you may think, as a man, that you should be able to tough things out—because you'll probably end up feeling a failure as well as scared.
➲ Start talking. It might not be easy, but sharing your fears and concerns could help make them feel easier to deal with. Consider seeing a counselor or joining a support group to meet other people with the same or similar illnesses.

Start taking control

Thirty years ago, the medical profession expected patients passively to put up with whatever was judged to be in their best interests. You took your medicine—even if you weren't exactly sure what it was—and simply hoped for the best. Although some doctors might still like to return to the days when a grateful public saw them as distant, all-powerful gods, most now believe that patients should be much more involved in the management of their condition. The idea is that the patient who feels in control—or 'empowered'—is much more likely to do well.

Key tips:

➲ Find out the facts. The more you know about your condition, the less frightening it will probably seem; the reality is unlikely to be as bad as the fears your mind is capable of generating at three in the morning. Contact organizations that offer advice, support, and information to people affected by your illness.

➲ Don't blame yourself for being ill. Whatever the cause of your health problem—and it's often hard to be sure exactly why illness strikes—it's important to remember that you never intended to become unwell. Rather than sinking into self-recrimination, try to focus on what you can do to recover.

➲ Eat well. Changing your diet could help improve your condition—a low-fat diet is important in treating heart disease, for example, and weight loss due to ill-health may need to be tackled by a special high-calorie diet— as well as making you feel as if you're generally taking better care of yourself.

➲ Exercise. Again, this could be a part of your treatment (if you're recovering from a heart attack, for example) or you could get moving simply because it makes you feel good. You should ask your doctor what level of exercise is appropriate: rushing off to the gym and humping weights for an hour might not be advisable if you're still recovering from major surgery.

➲ Relax. Meditation, massage, and yoga are excellent stressbusters. One recent study found the level of pain following major abdominal surgery can be significantly reduced by using a simple relaxation exercise and/or listening to soothing music.

➲ Stay in touch. There's increasing evidence that people are much more likely to recover from serious illnesses if they have a good network of social relationships.

➲ Develop a positive mental attitude. There's good evidence that feeling optimistic and hopeful are important factors in recovery from a range of serious illnesses. Becoming permanently pessimistic or apathetic isn't likely to help you get better.

These suggestions could help:

○ List (and regularly remind yourself of) all the big reasons why it's important for you to get better (e.g. 'I want to see my children grow up,' 'I want to write that novel I've been thinking about for years').

○ Set yourself specific, manageable goals not directly connected with your health (e.g. learning a foreign language or a musical instrument, doing volunteer work, getting promoted at work, decorating your house).

○ Think about yourself as a 'survivor' or 'someone living with "x" illness' rather than as a 'patient,' 'ex-patient,' or (worst of all) a 'victim'. Adopting the mental outlook of a survivor can help you become an active participant in the healing process. The victim mode is passive, however, and implicitly hands over the responsibility for recovery to someone else.

○ Watch films and videos. Stories about people who triumph over adversity could prove encouraging and inspiring. Tastes will vary, but *Chariots of Fire* and *Gandhi* are worth trying. Optimistic visions of the future might help, too, such as *Star Trek: The Next Generation*. And don't forget comedy: in a now well-known case, an American editor, Norman Cousins, claims he recovered from a disabling spinal condition by watching funny films. Dr Patch Adams also uses humor as a central plank of treatment at the Gesundheit Institute medical center in the USA.

○ Open a book. You might also get inspiration from reading about how other people have overcome seemingly impossible odds. Brian Keenan's account of his time as a hostage in Beirut, *An Evil Cradling*, is an outstanding example. Autobiographical accounts of dealing with illness could also help: try Michael Korda's *Man to Man*, an account of surviving prostate cancer.

○ Improve your environment. Hospitals are discovering that simple steps like having art on the walls can significantly improve patients' recovery rates. You can also create a more esthetically pleasing atmosphere at home by sticking up some posters or cuttings from magazines; vases of fresh flowers can also make a big difference.

○ See your illness as a teacher. It's easy to see a health problem as simply something to be fought against. But it can also help to see an illness as a process to learn from. Many people find it provides a valuable opportunity to re-evaluate their lives. They might realize that their previous lifestyle was unsustainable or ultimately unfulfilling; indeed, it might have contributed directly to their illness. They could decide to make key changes, perhaps working fewer hours, moving to a more pleasant environment, or spending more time with friends and family. It's become a bit of a cliché, but men often say that the experience of serious illness completely changes their priorities and that it enables them for the first time to discover the true value of life's everyday pleasures.

○ Try 'mental imagery.' Practice an exercise in which you visualize the process through which your body heals itself from illness. Although you need to discover the imagery that suits you best, it might help to see germs or diseased cells as a small, weak, and defenceless enemy being effortlessly destroyed by the superior firepower of your defender cells. If that feels too violent, try imagining yourself as a gardener steadily removing small, rotten weeds and replacing them with large, healthy, vibrant flowers. Christopher Reeve, the actor who played Superman in four films, says he found it helpful to use imagery shortly after he became severely disabled following a horse-riding accident. 'Someone, a stranger, had sent me a picture postcard of a Mayan temple in Mexico, the Pyramid of Quetzalcoatl,' he writes in his autobiography *Still Me*. 'There were hundreds of steps leading to the top. And above the temple were blue sky and clouds. I taped this postcard to the bottom of the [hospital] monitor, where it was always in view. I let it become a metaphor for the future. Even as I watched all those sobering numbers on the screen, I began to imagine myself climbing those steps, one at a time, until finally I would reach the top and go into the sky.'

Consider complementary therapies

Complementary, or alternative, therapies are no longer the preserve just of weird hippies or wealthy eccentrics. Many are being researched by mainstream scientists, and some are beginning to be offered by orthodox medical practitioners. The US National Institute of Health has already judged acupuncture to have a useful role in the treatment of back pain, asthma, headaches, addictions, and chemotherapy-related nausea. Far from being critical of patients who try different approaches to healing, many doctors now want them to receive the best possible package of treatments; increasingly, health professionals are talking not of 'complementary' and 'orthodox' medicine but of 'integrated' medicine.

Complementary therapies offer two key benefits. First, they treat you holistically; in other words, a practitioner will normally focus on all aspects of your life and how they might be affecting your well-being. Unlike with orthodox medicine, you're not seen as just having a defective body part that requires specific treatment. Secondly, you'll

THE SCIENCE BIT

○ A study of 122 men who'd had a heart attack found that, after eight years, 21 of the 25 most pessimistic men had died; of the 25 most optimistic, just six had died. Mental outlook proved a better predictor of survival than any medical risk factor, including the severity of the first heart attack, cholesterol levels, or blood pressure.

○ Another study of over 300 coronary artery by-pass patients found those who felt optimistic were 23 per cent less likely than pessimists to be readmitted to hospital within six months of their surgery.

○ An investigation of 57 people paralyzed by spinal injuries found that those with most hope gained greater levels of physical mobility than other patients with similar injuries who felt less hopeful.

○ Other research shows that the greater your belief that you can return to a normal life after a heart attack, the more likely you are to do so.

almost certainly get more time with your practitioner than you ever will with your doctor. This gives you an opportunity to discuss all your concerns about your health problems.

Because complementary therapies can differ as much from each other as they do from orthodox medicine, it's impossible to pass judgement on them as a whole. To be either for or against complementary medicine is as absurd as being for or against television. There are effective and ineffective therapies just as there are good and bad programs. What matters is to be able to pick the therapies that are most likely to help you.

Key tips:

➲ Consider a therapy that makes sense to you. If you have little or no confidence in a therapy, then it's much less likely to be of benefit. You might prefer a therapy for which there's considerable scientific support (e.g. acupuncture or herbalism) than one for which there's little or no conclusive evidence of effectiveness (e.g. crystal therapy or reflexology). Alternatively, you could be more willing to accept an approach simply because you feel it makes strong intuitive sense.

➲ Be realistic about your goals. If you're looking for a cure for cancer, you're almost certainly going to be disappointed. But if you want a means of reducing pain, anxiety, or stress, or relief from the side-effects or chemotherapy, then several complementary therapies could probably help.

➲ Choose a therapy you'll be comfortable with. If you're needle-phobic, for instance, acupuncture probably isn't for you; if you don't want to be touched by a stranger, avoid massage; if you're not prepared to invest a significant amount of time, you're unlikely to benefit much from meditation or yoga.

➲ Make sure your practitioner is qualified. You probably wouldn't hand over your car to someone who wasn't a trained mechanic; don't do the same with your body. Try contacting a national organization that represents the therapy you're interested in and ask to be sent a list of accredited practitioners in your area.

➲ Discuss any complementary therapy you're interested in with your doctor before you start—you need to be sure it won't interfere with any other treatment you're receiving.

Take it easy

Most health problems require a period of rest and relaxation in order for healing to occur. It's no coincidence that you tend to feel tired when you're unwell: the body's resources are focused on tackling your illness, not getting you ready to commute to work or run a marathon. But many men find it difficult to take time off and put their feet up; if you've been brought up to believe a man's role is to be active and vigorous, it can be hard to lie in bed all day watching endless repeats of *Chicago Hope* and *ER*. While staying active might make you feel as if you still have some control over your life, it could seriously delay your recovery.

Key tips:
➲ Ask your doctor exactly what level of rest you need. It may be that you can in fact be more active than you think.

➲ Listen to your body. Although you may not be used to being guided by your body's needs, how tired you feel can be a useful pointer to how much you need to rest.

➲ Think ahead. Remind yourself that if you rest properly now you stand a greater chance of being more active later. See it as a worthwhile trade-off.

➲ Remain stimulated. Even if you do have to rest for long periods, it doesn't mean you have to shut your brain down. Consider what you'd like to read, rent videos of films you've always wanted to see, listen to the radio, get hold of audio books, compile a stock of your favorite music.

➲ Keep in touch. It can get lonely resting all day, so keep in touch with friends and family by telephone and e-mail. Ask people to visit you—or at least say 'yes, please' when they offer. You may feel embarrassed or even ashamed to see people when you're feeling sick, but you should remember that feeling connected to other people has significant healing qualities.

➲ Forget about work. Although you might be worried about the consequences of taking time off work, returning too soon is unlikely to help your recuperation. If you're not completely better when you do return, you may need to consider working fewer hours or temporarily switching to less stressful work.

➲ Forget about those household repairs (however essential). If you're too ill to work, you're also too ill to paint the living room or build a new patio.

➲ Let other people care for you. If you're lying in bed with a broken leg, recovering from flu, cancer, or depression, or generally feeling weak and rotten because of any other health problem, you're unlikely to be able to get by on your own, however much you might want to. You may well need some help

LEADING COMPLEMENTARY THERAPIES

(Ω = poor evidence; $\Omega\Omega\Omega\Omega\Omega$ = very good evidence)

Acupuncture

What Is It? Needles are inserted at key points in the skin to 'rebalance' the body's energy flow.

Does it work? $\Omega\Omega\Omega\Omega\Omega$

What is it particularly suitable for? Pain relief, back pain, asthma, depression, nausea, high blood pressure, digestive problems, stress.

Aromatherapy

What is it? Essential oils (e.g. lavender, peppermint, rosemary) with healing properties are massaged into the body, inhaled, or added to bath water.

Does it work? $\Omega\Omega$

What is it particularly suitable for? Stress-related problems, skin complaints, digestive disorders, asthma.

LEADING COMPLEMENTARY THERAPIES

Chiropractic

What is it? A system of manipulating the skeletal structure to restore the body's natural harmony.

Does it work? ∩∩∩∩∩

What is it particularly suitable for? Spine, neck, and muscle problems, headaches, migraines, digestive disorders.

Crystal therapy

What is it? Crystals are believed to possess healing energies which are released when held on or near the body.

Does it work? ∩

What is it particularly suitable for? It's probably only worth trying (for any condition) if you're convinced it will work—there's a chance you could benefit from a 'placebo effect'.

Herbalism

What is it? Herbs restore the body's ability to heal itself and can, like conventional drugs, have a direct effect.

Does it work? ∩∩∩∩∩

What is it particularly suitable for? Most illnesses.

Homeopathy

What is it? A minute amount of a substance that would produce the patient's symptoms acts to stimulate the body's self-healing abilities.

Does it work? ∩∩∩

What is it particularly suitable for? Most illnesses.

LEADING COMPLEMENTARY THERAPIES

Hypnotherapy

What is it? The patient is hypnotized and open to suggestion.

Does it work? ∩∩∩∩

What is it particularly suitable for? Pain relief, fears and phobias, stress, anxiety, depression, insomnia, addictions, digestive disorders.

Massage

What is it? Your skin and muscles are stroked and kneaded.

Does it work? ∩∩∩∩

What is it particularly suitable for? Stress-related problems, muscle and joint problems (including back pain), pain relief, depression, anxiety.

Meditation

What is it? It involves withdrawing from external reality, becoming deeply relaxed, and achieving increased mental clarity.

Does it work? ∩∩∩∩∩

What is it particularly suitable for? Stress, anxiety, high blood pressure, insomnia, addictions, headaches, pain relief, a depressed immune system.

Osteopathy

What is it? Massage and manipulation are used to improve joint mobility, relax stiff muscles, and restore balanced movement to the body.

Does it work? ∩∩∩∩∩

What is it particularly suitable for? Back and neck pain, joint pain, headaches, insomnia, depression, digestive disorders.

LEADING COMPLEMENTARY THERAPIES

Reflexology

What is it?	Foot massage stimulates specific areas of the body to promote healing.
Does it work?	◌◌
What is it particularly suitable for?	Stress, anxiety, insomnia, back pain, constipation.

Shiatsu

What is it?	Similar to acupuncture, except that massage is used instead of needles.
Does it work?	◌◌
What is it particularly suitable for?	Stress, back and neck pain, headaches.

Yoga

What is it?	A range of body postures and breathing techniques tone the body, oxygenate the blood, and strengthen the spine.
Does it work?	◌◌◌◌◌
What is it particularly suitable for?	Stress, back pain, fatigue, headaches, depression, asthma, hay fever, digestive disorders.

from a wide range of people. There's your doctor, of course, and nurses if you're in hospital. At home, you may need the support of a professional carer or you might rely on your partner, family, or friends for meals, shopping, and housework. It can be difficult for a man to feel dependent on others, but learning to accept help is an important part of getting better.

The final curtain

The prospect of dying is almost inevitably frightening; it can make us feel chillingly alone and abandoned. However powerful we might be, and however much money we might have, we're ultimately incapable of preventing death, the final equalizer. Death is largely beyond our control, a simple fact that escapes those men who

WHAT WILL I EXPERIENCE WHEN I DIE?

No one knows for sure, for the obvious reason that people who have died can't tell us. But it is known that many people who very nearly die later report a range of similar apparently mystical sensations. These are known, appropriately enough, as Near Death Experiences (or NDEs). They typically involve an out-of-body experience, such as looking down on oneself dying, or simply a feeling of deep peace followed by a sense of floating up through a tunnel toward a bright light. Assuming that NDEs don't really represent the transition to an after-life, one possibility is that they are hallucinations caused by the effects of medication or a lack of oxygen reaching the brain. The fact that many people tend to believe they are rising to heaven could reflect the enduring power of these images in even a secular, rational society. But the frequency with which these sorts of images are experienced can offer us some reassurance that nearing the moment of death may not be the terrifying experience many of us dread.

spend fortunes having their bodies frozen so they can be resurrected when the medical technology of the future can cure whatever they died of. Since very few of us want to die, it might at first seem glib to speak of a 'good death,' the kind of passing that we feel we've come to terms with. But facing the ultimate unknown with a degree of acceptance is surely preferable to viewing it simply with fear and foreboding. It doesn't mean that we've given up the will to live, but it could relieve a great deal of stress and anxiety.

Key tips:
- Accept the possibility of death. We may die sooner than we'd like, but it's an unalterable fact that we're all mortal; indeed, every living thing on the planet at some point has to die. Death is an integral part of the process of life.
- Understand that death isn't the end of us. Whether or not you believe in an after-life, there's no doubt that we'll be remembered by those who knew us. We have an existence that continues beyond the inscriptions on a tombstone.
- Parts of us will live on. It's a scientific fact that much of the matter that makes us up will eventually nourish and become part of the structure of plants and other animals. This process will continue until the end of time (and, of course, time is incomprehensibly boundless).

➲ Understand the process of death. However we die, it's unlikely to be the sudden, instantaneous, and violent death we see every day on television or at the movies. Most deaths occur as the result of a progressive illness. While this may cause pain and suffering over a long period, it also enables us to prepare for the possibility of dying.

➲ Take pride in your achievements. No life is without its accomplishments; you needn't have become chief of a multinational oil company to have lived a life of value. Reflect on every aspect of your life, including your relationships, your creativity, your humor, and your work. To get a perspective on your significance, watch Frank Capra's film *It's a Wonderful Life*. It reveals just how much impact one man's life can have on his family and community and how big a hole is left by his death.

➲ Mend important but damaged relationships. The prospect of death can make the issues that once bitterly divided us from others seem trivial. Feeling at peace with those who have been or are significant in your life can be extremely important.

➲ Sort out the practicalities. Make sure you have drawn up an up-to-date will and left clear instructions about your care should you become too ill to make decisions for yourself. Decide what sort of funeral and burial or cremation you would prefer.

➲ Keep talking. When people know they are approaching death they tend to move through a series of psychological stages. They start by being unable to accept that they will really die. This is followed by anger, an attempt to 'bargain' (e.g. promising to some higher power that 'If I live until my birthday I will donate my body to medical science'), depression, and, finally, acceptance. Most people don't move through the stages in one direction: they can go backward and forward and even experience two or more of the stages simultaneously. But many find it much easier to reach the final stage of acceptance if they can find a way of communicating their feelings about death. Because this can be distressing to people who are close to you, it may well be easier to talk to a counselor.

➲ Enjoy yourself. Whether you've got two months or two years to live, try not to become so obsessed with death that you forget you're still alive. It could help to continue to take part in experiences that are satisfying, enriching, and give you the feeling of having lived a full and good life.

CHAPTER 15

HEY, GOOD-LOOKING:
FEELING GREAT ABOUT YOUR BODY

Men increasingly want to look and feel good. It's no longer possible simply to dismiss us all as overweight slobs with bad breath and dirty fingernails. In the last 20 years there's been nothing less than a revolution in the way many of us take care of our bodies: we're spending more time working out, paying greater attention to our diet, beginning to take personal grooming seriously, and buying an ever-expanding range of men's health and fitness magazines. Most of us may never look like the lean, muscular and stereotypically handsome guys on the covers but we're more likely than ever to be doing our best with what we've got.

At the same time, however, many of us are feeling increasingly self-conscious about our appearance. Even though we're spending more time in the gym and the bathroom, we're still not sure it's enough. Almost six out of 10 men say they've been depressed by their physique and 50 per cent feel pressure from the media to have a perfect body, according to a survey of 1500 men by a UK men's health magazine. Abdominal fat is the biggest concern: 56 per cent worry about love handles and 54 per cent about a beer belly. Some men now feel compelled to diet to the point where they develop anorexia or bulimia; others attempt to achieve the same result through compulsive exercise. Ever-greater numbers of men are also seeking instant rejuvenation through cosmetic surgery or are using anabolic steroids to develop massive muscles.

The challenge many of us now face is to find a way of taking good care of our bodies, and to feel positive about how we look, without becoming obsessed with achieving an unrealistic level of physical perfection. Although this might feel difficult, the good news is that there are many practical steps we can take to enable us to develop a much more positive body image.

Here's looking at you

There's no magic way for a man to start feeling great about his body. It's not simply a matter of wearing an Armani suit, exercising, and dieting until he's acquired a six-pack or asking a cosmetic surgeon to transform him into a George Clooney lookalike. Becoming comfortable with one's body image involves a rather more subtle process.

○ Accept that you're probably never going to look like Richard Gere, Jean-Claude van Damme or Leonardo di Caprio. Like it or loathe it, genes are the biggest determinant of your physical appearance and you're stuck for life with the ones you've been born with. If you're an 'ectomorph' (with a light, lean body), for example, you're very unlikely to be able to develop the muscle mass of an 'endomorph' like Arnold Schwarzenegger (a man with a naturally large, muscular build). Similarly, if you've lost most of your hair, you're never going to get it back, no matter how much money you spend on lotions and hair transplants. If you believe you can somehow over-ride the effects of your genetic inheritance, you're setting yourself up for failure.
○ Understand that your body image can be affected by a wide range of factors outside your direct control.
○ Media images can have a big impact, according to research at Manchester Metropolitan University in the UK. Psychologists there discovered that men reacted to magazine photographs of male models by feeling less satisfied with their own bodies and experiencing lowered self-esteem.
○ Your body image may have been affected by taunts from other children in the school playground or hurtful comments from a partner or family members. Children in particular often don't hesitate to mock each other's physical differences. Simply wearing spectacles can make a child a figure of fun in the eyes of his peers. Feelings of ugliness you experienced even 20 years ago can easily live on, even if you now look very different.
○ If you belong to an ethnic minority, you may well have been exposed to negative, racist images about your people's appearance that permeate the culture you've grown up in. It's difficult to resist eventually believing that some of these may be true, a process known as 'internalization'. In most Western countries, you're also constantly exposed to a media that perpetuates the idea that the 'ideal' man is white and has sharp, chiseled features and straight hair.

Becoming more aware of these influences can enable you to make a more realistic assessment of your appearance.

DO SOME MEN HAVE 'ATTRACTIVE' GENES?

You've probably seen reports of research suggesting that women are biologically programmed to be attracted to men with certain facial features and body shapes. Some studies suggest that women are more likely to desire men with symmetrical bodies or feminine faces. One researcher claims that women prefer a more feminine face except for the time each month when they're most likely to become pregnant; then they're more likely to be attracted to stereotypically masculine faces.

The problem with this research, apart from the fact that it's somewhat contradictory, is that it's mostly based on showing women photographs of men's faces and bodies. Even if it's accurate, it ignores the fact that in real life women are attracted to men for many reasons besides their physical appearance—a sense of humor, emotional maturity, even money or power can all be much more important. Looking conventionally attractive might make a difference in the first nanosecond of meeting someone, but if a man behaves like a dork he's quickly going to offend more than a woman's sight.

○ One of the secrets of acquiring a positive body image is to develop the kind of relationship with your body that feels right for you rather than attempting to replicate the media's idea of the perfect physique.

Key tips:
➲ Acknowledge that there's more than one way of looking good. Tom Cruise and Robert Redford are undoubtedly attractive to many, but so is the French actor, Gerard Depardieu. During his time in President Nixon's White House, Henry Kissinger was widely held to be one of the sexiest men in Washington. In other words, it's possible to be middle-aged, overweight, bespectacled, and not at all like a stereotypically handsome hunk and still be considered extremely desirable. If you're unconvinced, think about your female friends. Do you really believe they can't be attractive or sexy unless they happen to look like Sharon Stone or Pamela Anderson?
➲ Reconsider your role models. Do you still secretly want to look like the football players, movie stars, and other men you worshiped when you were a teenager? Perhaps it's time to acquire some new heroes with more rounded personalities. They don't have to be public figures; men

known only within your community may be perfectly able to provide the inspiration and lead you're looking for. But if you are stuck for someone, how about Nelson Mandela? He's a man respected by millions for his humanity, integrity, wisdom, and humor, not because he spends his spare time in the gym attempting to create the perfect body.

○ See your body as a whole. When you think about your body, the chances are that you almost always focus on what you're unhappy with. You probably ignore those parts that are okay or which, if you spent a few moments thinking about them, you'd realize are actually in pretty good shape. It's important not just to consider the obvious bits—the hair (or lack of it) on your head, your nose, ears, chest, abdomen, buttocks, and penis. Remember also to notice your eyes, lips, teeth, neck, body hair, arms, hands, fingers, legs, knees, ankles, feet, and toes.

○ Appreciate that your body image is affected by far more than your physical appearance. If you have a good sex life, feel loved and respected by others, are physically fit or satisfied and fulfilled at work or by your hobbies, the odds are you'll feel better about most aspects of your life, including how you look. Rather than focusing on changing your body size and shape, you might end up with a more positive body image if you considered how you can boost your overall sense of satisfaction with life. This could mean paying more attention to exercise, the quality of your relationships, your work, your emotional health, and your stress levels.

○ Ask yourself whether changing your body really would make the difference to your life that you hope for. Some men find that when their lives seem unfulfilled or out of control, they can end up becoming preoccupied with changing their body shape; they can feel as if it's just about the last area over which they can make a difference or exercise some real control. Other men can convince themselves that developing a firmer, more muscular body would give them a stronger sense of being manly or masculine. Do you believe, for instance, that achieving a goal like a flat stomach or regaining your hair will somehow solve one or more unconnected problems? If you have an exaggerated view of what changing your body shape might achieve, you may well need to look for another solution to whatever's worrying you.

○ Enjoy your body. You're more likely to feel positive about your body if you're able to see it as a source of enjoyment and pleasure rather than an object that simply carries you around or that you regularly drag to the gym for an exhausting workout.

DO YOU REALLY WANT A SIX-PACK?

The men's fitness magazines relentlessly instruct us how to 'Lose that gut' and 'Get killer abs now,' reflecting the fact that men's abdomens are supposed to be as flat, and as hard, as a brick wall.

But before you rush off to the gym, remember this:

○ A six-pack stomach won't make you healthier. Your abdominal muscles probably won't be visible unless your body fat level falls to less than 10 per cent of your body weight. This is far below the desirable healthy range for men (14–17 per cent).
○ Your diet will be boring. To get your body fat levels down, you'll probably have to make sure that no more than 15 per cent of your calories come from fat (that's half of the World Health Organization recommended level). To achieve it, you'll not only have to double-check everything you eat but you'll also suffer from serious taste deprivation.
○ It'll take hours and hours. Most experts agree that two or three vigorous 20–30 minute aerobic workouts each week are enough to create a good level of fitness. To achieve a six-pack, you'll probably have to set aside at least another four or five hours a week for exercise. This means you'll have a lot less time for whatever else you enjoy doing in your spare time.
○ A washboard won't make you happy. If you believe that achieving a six-pack is the key to personal success and satisfaction then you're almost certainly deluding yourself.
○ You could be wasting your time. Your genetic make-up will not only affect how easily you can acquire a six-pack, it will also determine whether you can develop one at all. Your biology may mean that you'll never do better than a two-pack, however hard you try.

Key tips:
➲ Get sensual. That means finding ways of deriving pleasure from body contact that isn't erotic or sexual. Try massaging your own body with a hand or body lotion, sharing a massage with a partner, or having the occasional professional massage.
➲ Be sexual. Masturbation or sex with a partner aren't compulsory, but they can be a wonderful physical (as well as emotional) experience.

Explore the possibilities, and, if you have a sexual problem, get expert advice and help.

⊃ Exercise. If you don't do much or any, consider making it a regular part of your life. Walking is a great way to start. If you're already exercising frequently, don't stick to the same old workouts but experiment with new activities. If you normally cycle, try running, rowing, swimming, or roller-blading as alternatives. If you enjoy competitive sports, try something different: if you're a regular squash player, how about the occasional game of tennis or badminton? Whatever type of exercise you take, try to see it not just as a means of getting fit; it's important also to enjoy how it feels when you push your body beyond its normal limits. (See Chapter 4 for some more ideas about exercise.)

⊃ Try Eastern systems of movement. Yoga and t'ai chi stretch the body in ways that are both disciplined and relaxed (see page 52). Qigong (pronounced 'chee-gong') is another similar system combining movement, breathing techniques, and meditation.

⊃ Dance. This isn't only great exercise, it's also a way of learning new ways of experiencing your body and expressing yourself.

○ Respect your body. It's the only one you've got, so it makes sense to look after it. And the more you take care of your body, the more you're also likely to feel positive about it. Finding time to relax, eating a healthy diet, being a healthy weight, drinking alcohol moderately, and not smoking could all make a big difference. It might also be worth finding new ways to pamper yourself: try leisurely hot baths, saunas, and hot tubs. If you shave, take it seriously rather than tearing your face to shreds with any old razor and soap.

The bald facts

Most men eventually lose all or most of their hair—and the majority of them hate that fact. Thinning normally begins in the late teens, and by the age of 30, 50 per cent of men have a visibly receding hairline and 30 per cent are thinning on top. The most common cause is a condition known as androgenetic alopecia (or male pattern baldness), caused by the interaction of baldness genes with the male sex hormones. White men are particularly badly affected: they are four times more likely than black men to go bald prematurely. Contrary to popular belief, there's no link between hair loss and sexual potency.

A CLOSE SHAVE

The perfect shave is probably unachievable outside the fantasy world of razor advertisements, but these tips should help:

○ Wet those whiskers. Warm water causes facial hair to expand and soften, making it easier to cut.
○ Get in a lather. Shaving foam, cream, or gel holds in the heat and moisture and contains lubricants that provide a smoother shave. Special formulations are available for sensitive skin.
○ Shave with the grain and in one direction. The shave may not be as close this way, but the cut hairs are much less likely to grow back into the skin.
○ Don't stretch. Pulling the skin taut risks cutting the hairs below the skin surface, increasing the likelihood of ingrowing hairs.
○ Keep it clean. Rinse the razor with hot water several times during shaving. Change the blade regularly (if it is starting to draw blood it has to go) and always use clean, unshared towels.
○ If wet shaving irritates the skin, try an electric razor.

There are two drugs—minoxidil and finasteride—that can often halt the decline, or even stimulate some regrowth, but they have to be taken indefinitely. Scalp surgery is a possibility, but it's expensive and not always effective; if hair loss continues, moreover, it may have to be repeated. A wig is a final option, but a high-quality hairpiece is not only costly but also cannot totally eliminate the fear of exposure following a sudden gust of strong wind. Perhaps men's best long-term solution is to try to come to terms with their hair loss.

Although hair is still associated with physical attractiveness, baldness is definitely becoming more fashionable. More balding men are now rejecting the comb-over strategy and having their hair cut short all over. Icons like Bruce Willis, Sean Connery, and Jack Nicholson appear happy to display visibly receding hairlines. Anthony Edwards, the star of the US television series *ER*, is a baldie; so too is Patrick Stewart, who plays Jean-Luc Picard, the captain of the Starship *Enterprise*. Bald liberation is even on the agenda, led by the Bald-headed Men of America. They believe a man should be judged by what goes on in his head, not on top of it, and stand for his right to be proud of every single hair he no longer has.

Words of warning

Some men's pursuit of the perfect body can cause serious problems.

○ Cosmetic surgery. Up to 40 per cent of clients in some UK clinics are now male. The options routinely available range from face lifts and nose reshaping to penis lengthening and even the insertion of silicone pectoral muscles in the chest. It seems men are no longer obliged to accept passively the legacy of their genes; they can now ask medical science to put right whatever they believe nature has got wrong.

COSMETIC SURGERY: THE PROS AND CONS

Pros	Cons
A relatively quick process: you can lose more fat from your abdomen in an hour's surgery than in two months of eating a low-fat diet.	The surgery is painful and carries a risk of infection and other side-effects.
	It's expensive.
Surgery can provide the 'kick start' some people need to change their lifestyle.	It's not always a permanent solution: unless you change your lifestyle as well, problems like a large abdomen will eventually return. Face lifts or hair transplants may need to be repeated every few years.
Some changes—e.g. changing the shape of your ears or nose—can't be achieved in any other way.	
Many patients experience a significant rise in self-esteem after their surgery.	The results may not be as good as you hoped and may even look worse than before. One study of men seeking medical help after penile cosmetic surgery found that 50 per cent needed a further operation and only eight per cent felt their penis was actually longer.

AM I BIG ENOUGH?

Psychologists have recently identified a condition known as 'muscle dysmorphia.' It occurs when a bodybuilder or an athlete has a totally false view of his body shape. Typically, he'll believe he's weak and puny even though, in reality, he's large and muscle-bound. Someone who suffers from this problem will become fixated on his body, exercise excessively, sacrifice relationships and a career in order to spend more time at the gym, and be much more likely to use anabolic steroids. A man who's convinced of his physical inadequacy can't be persuaded he's wrong by rational argument. The best treatment is counseling, although some psychiatrists have also found anti-depressants effective.

Anyone considering cosmetic surgery should not only make sure they see a fully qualified and experienced surgeon at a reputable clinic but also consider independent counseling before signing on the dotted line. Many men have unrealistic expectations of what surgery can achieve—even when it goes well—and may remain unhappy with their appearance if they haven't tackled the fundamental cause of their negative body image.

○ Compulsive exercise. Although exercise is undoubtedly good for health and the development of a positive body image, some men actually become addicted. One theory is that they become hooked on the 'high' generated by the natural 'feel-good' opiates (endorphins) produced in the brain. Whatever the reason, compulsive exercisers start suffering withdrawal symptoms if they're prevented from working out (see page 98). Some men feel driven by their addiction to exercise even when they're injured or ill; this could have serious effects on their health and their ability to continue exercising in the long-term. Other signs of exercise addiction include neglecting other aspects of life in order to spend more time exercising, feeling tired all the time, and becoming obsessional about food. Exercise addiction is difficult to self-treat, and if you suspect you're affected by it your best bet is to see a counselor.
○ Anabolic steroids. When combined with resistance exercise, these hormonal drugs can certainly increase muscle mass, but at a heavy price. They can damage the liver and kidneys, increase blood pressure, reduce sperm production, enlarge men's breasts, and cause depression during

the period of withdrawal from the drugs. Steroids often cause mood swings, too, including increased aggression (so-called 'roid rage'). If you use steroids, your first priority must be to minimize the risk by always using clean injecting equipment. If you decide you want to stop but can't, you could contact a specialist drugs agency for advice. You may also need counseling to help you to think about why it feels so important to develop large muscles.

○ Eating disorders. Anorexia, bulimia, binge-eating—you might think these affect only women, but 10 per cent of all those with an eating disorder are male. It's hard to recognize if you have a disorder, but the symptoms to look out for include:

➲ An intense fear of gaining weight.

➲ Having a distorted view of your body image—you may well believe you're overweight even though you're actually underweight.

➲ You believe your whole life will be better once you've got the body shape you want.

➲ You don't enjoy eating as a social activity and prefer to eat alone so that other people can't see or comment on your food.

➲ You feel as if food, eating, and your weight completely dominate your life.

➲ You regularly and uncontrollably binge-eat, perhaps followed by vomiting, using laxatives or excessive exercise to try and compensate.

➲ You feel as if your level of exercise must always be increasing and that you mustn't miss out on it.

➲ You experience health problems as a result of an inadequate diet.

If you believe you have an eating disorder, you will almost certainly need professional help from a counselor with experience of this problem.

CHAPTER 16

WHAT'S UP, DOC?

THE ESSENTIAL ENCYCLOPEDIA
OF MEN'S HEALTH PROBLEMS

Let's say you've developed an unusual ache or lump you can't explain. What do you do? One option is to try to ignore it and hope it goes away. Another is to convince yourself that it can't really be anything serious. While there's obviously a good chance that you've got only a minor problem, you could be ignoring something potentially much more dangerous, so both these strategies put you at risk. Although your best bet is always to seek medical advice for any worry you have about your health, it's also useful to find out more for yourself. That's where this chapter can help. It will enable you to make sense of any symptoms you might develop and tell you how best to deal with them.

This chapter doesn't cover every health problem a man might suffer from. Some, like stress and depression, are dealt with elsewhere. There simply isn't the space to deal with many other general health problems such as flu, acne, or hemorrhoids; for more information about these, you'll need to consult one of the many excellent and widely available health reference books. This chapter focuses on health problems that affect only men. But because heart disease and all forms of cancer are so important, some brief information has been included about how to prevent them, the main symptoms to look out for, and the most common treatments.

CANCER

WHAT ARE THE MAIN SYMPTOMS?
- A change in bowel or bladder habits.
- A persistent sore throat, nagging cough, or hoarseness.
- Unusual bleeding or discharge.
- Thickening or lump in the testicles or elsewhere.
- Persistent indigestion.
- Difficulty in swallowing.
- Obvious change in size or bleeding of a mole.

All of these symptoms can also be caused by minor or benign (i.e. non-cancerous) health problems. But because some cancers can grow quickly, it's vital to seek medical advice as soon as you think you might have a problem. The sooner treatment can begin, the greater your chances of a full recovery.
See page 234 for more details of penile cancer, page 243 for prostate cancer, and page 255 for testicular cancer.

WHAT'S THE RISK?
- Considerable. About one in four of us will develop some form of cancer.
- The risk increases greatly with age: it's low below 30, roughly doubles between 30 and 40 and then doubles again in each of the following decades.

WHAT CAUSES IT?
- Most cancers are the result of a combination of genetic susceptibility and carcinogenic (or cancer-causing) triggers such as certain foods (e.g. fat), tobacco, alcohol, sunlight, some viruses, and chemicals in environmental pollutants.

HOW CAN I PREVENT IT?
- Reduce or eliminate exposure to carcinogens, especially tobacco.
- Eat more fruit and vegetables.
- Take regular exercise.
- Cope better with stress.
- Check yourself regularly for any of the early signs of cancer. If you're over 40, discuss with your doctor the value of regular screening for bowel and prostate cancers.

WHAT ARE THE MAIN TREATMENTS?
○ Surgery is normally used to remove the main site of the tumor.
○ Radiotherapy and chemotherapy are often also used to destroy cancer cells that may have spread to other areas.

WHAT'S THE OUTLOOK?
○ Cancer definitely isn't an automatic death sentence. Almost half of all cancers are now cured completely, and the survival rates for most are steadily improving.

HEART DISEASE

WHAT ARE THE MAIN SYMPTOMS?
○ You may not know you've got heart disease until you develop the symptoms of either angina or a heart attack. These include:
➲ Chest pain that feels like being squeezed or crushed. The pain usually starts in the center of the chest and can spread to the throat, upper jaw, back, and arms. The pain of a heart attack is usually severe; angina pain can range from mild to severe.
➲ The chest pain may be accompanied by nausea, vomiting, sweating, dizziness, breathlessness, or fainting.
➲ Angina pain usually starts when the heart is working harder—during physical activity, stress, or when the temperature is extreme—and will ease with rest. Heart attack pain can start at any time and doesn't ease with rest.

If you believe you could be having a heart attack, rest and call an ambulance immediately.

WHAT'S THE RISK?
○ Significant. Although death rates are now falling, one in three men dies of heart disease.

WHAT CAUSES IT?
○ Cholesterol-rich fatty deposits stick to the artery walls, causing them to narrow. Artery-blocking blood clots can also develop in these areas.
○ Smoking, a lack of exercise, high blood pressure, being overweight, and a diet high in saturated fat are also factors.
○ Some people have a genetic predisposition to heart disease.

HOW CAN I PREVENT IT?
- Eat a low-fat and low-salt diet with plenty of fruit and vegetables.
- Quit smoking.
- Control your weight.
- Have regular physical activity.
- Cope better with stress.
- Have regular blood-pressure checks. Consider regular cholesterol checks, too, especially if you smoke, are overweight, and have high blood pressure.

WHAT ARE THE MAIN TREATMENTS?
- There are several drug treatments available for both angina and heart attacks.
- Both angina and a heart attack can also be treated with a procedure that widens narrowed arteries or an artery by-pass operation.

WHAT'S THE OUTLOOK?
- If you adopt a healthy lifestyle there's a very good chance you'll go on to lead a long and active life.

INFERTILITY

WHAT ARE THE MAIN SYMPTOMS?
- There are no obvious signs. The best clue is if you and your partner are unable to conceive after one year of unprotected sexual intercourse. You will then need to have a semen analysis to see whether you have a fertility problem.

WHAT'S THE RISK?
- As many as one in 20 men may have a fertility problem.
- Among infertile couples, about 30–40 per cent of cases stem solely from the man, 30–40 per cent from the woman, and the remainder from both.

WHAT CAUSES IT?
- *A varicocele.* This is basically a varicose vein on a testicle (see page 257). It's thought a varicocele can heat up the testicle, affecting the sperm production process.
- *Injury to the testicles.* Being hit in the testicles is not only painful, it can also damage the sperm-producing cells.

WHAT IS INFERTILITY?

A man is usually considered to have a fertility problem if his so-called 'semen profile' doesn't meet certain minimum criteria. There should be at least two millilitres of total ejaculate, 20 million sperm per millilitre of semen, 50 per cent of the sperm should be motile (i.e. moving positively rather than aimlessly swimming around in circles), and 30 per cent should be of normal shape rather than malformed. Other relevant factors include the ability of the sperm cell to escape from the seminal fluid in which it was ejaculated, to penetrate the woman's cervical mucus and then the egg's outer covering. One of the single most reliable indicators of a man's ability to initiate a pregnancy is the ability of his sperm to penetrate specially prepared hamster eggs in a laboratory test.

○ *Hormonal problems.* Four key hormones are involved—follicle-stimulating hormone (FSH), luteinising hormone (LH), testosterone, and prolactin—and any imbalance can affect sperm production.
○ *Antibodies.* Sperm motility can be affected by antibodies produced as a result of previous or current genital infections, including chlamydia and gonorrhea (see page 185).
○ *Blocked tubes.* Infections such as epididymitis (see page 254) can leave a legacy of scarring which blocks the very fine tubes that carry sperm away from the testicles.
○ *Retrograde ejaculation.* A condition where the valve at the neck of the bladder fails to close just before ejaculation. This means that the semen flows into the bladder rather than out through the penis. It's caused by prostate surgery and other conditions that damage the nerves around the bladder.
○ *Undescended testicles.* About one per cent of baby boys have undescended testicles, and even though surgery can bring the testicles down into the scrotum, some men are left with testicles that don't function normally.
○ *Drug use.*
　➲ Smoking—it lowers the levels of a man's sex hormones so he produces fewer sperm. One study showed that the sperm of a man who smokes 20 a day are only half as likely as a non-smoker's to penetrate and fertilize his partner's egg.

➲ Regular heavy drinking—it can reduce the number of sperm and possibly also damage them. Men who knock back over five pints of beer a day (or equivalent amounts of alcohol) are about half as likely to have normal sperm production as men who consume two-and-a-half units or fewer.

➲ Anabolic steroids—they may help you look like Arnold Schwarzenegger but your testicles will shrink as fast as your muscles will grow.

➲ Very high doses of cannabis—over 10 joints a week might affect sperm production, although the evidence is inconclusive. Cocaine and opiate drugs like heroin may also cause fertility problems.

➲ Some medically prescribed drugs—some of the drugs used to treat depression, high blood pressure, cancer, peptic ulcers, and other conditions may cause problems. If you're concerned about your fertility, discuss alternatives with your doctor (but don't stop taking the drugs first).

○ *Heat.* To produce sperm efficiently, the testicles must be 4°C cooler than normal body temperature. If they're heated up too much for too long, sperm production can be affected. Culprits include:

➲ Hot working conditions (e.g. in a bakery or welding).

➲ Too much driving (the partners of men who drive for more than three hours a day take significantly longer to conceive).

➲ Tight underwear has for a long time been blamed for warming up the testicles but recent US research suggests this may not be the case. It found that men's testicles are actually no hotter in Y-fronts than boxers—in fact, the study found that scrotums in boxers are, on average, fractionally hotter (by 0.2°C) than those in briefs.

○ *Occupational hazards.* Men working with lead (used to make storage batteries and paints), radiation, pesticides, and solvents are at risk of damaging their reproductive health.

○ *Stress.* Research suggests that chronic day-to-day stress can affect your sperm count. In one study, the men experiencing the highest stress levels had one-third fewer sperm in their semen than the most relaxed men. These sperm were also likely to be less motile. Other studies show that stress such as bereavement—and even having to provide a semen sample for *in vitro* fertilization treatment—can also adversely affect a man's semen profile.

○ *Sexual dysfunctions.* Many men are normally fertile but can't fertilize their partner simply because they're unable to achieve a satisfactory erection or because they ejaculate before penetration.

WHAT ABOUT FALLING SPERM COUNTS?

Many scientists believe that sperm counts are declining rapidly. One key study concluded that average sperm counts across many countries halved between 1940 and 1990 (from 113 million per milliliter of semen to 66) and that the volume of semen ejaculated also fell from 3.4 ml to 2.75 ml. A study of men in Scotland also found that men born in the 1950s had higher sperm counts, and higher numbers of motile sperm, than men born in the 1970s. The most plausible explanation put forward so far for this fall in semen quality is environmental pollution: chemicals that mimic the effects of the female sex hormone estrogen, such as DDT, other pesticides, and PCBs (polychlorinated biphenyls, used in the manufacture of electrical appliances) are affecting males' reproductive organs while they still growing in their mothers' wombs.

This long-term decline probably hasn't yet had any significant effect on men's ability to have children, however. An average sperm count of 66 million is still well above the fertility threshold of 20 million, and in any event sperm counts and motility are not the sole determinants of male fertility. But there can be little doubt that if present trends continue, and average sperm counts fall below 20 million (as they will before the end of the 21st century), many more men will then start experiencing fertility problems.

HOW CAN I PREVENT IT?
○ Your best bet is to lead a healthy lifestyle. Quitting smoking and drinking moderately are probably the two most obvious strategies.
○ Practicing safer sex will reduce your chances of developing a sexually transmitted infection, and regular sexual health check-ups should ensure that any such infection is treated promptly.
○ Avoid hot baths and saunas.
○ Find ways of coping better with stress.
○ If your work exposes you to potential risks, ensure health and safety regulations are strictly observed.

WHAT ARE THE MAIN TREATMENTS?
○ Make lifestyle changes which may help to improve your fertility (see above). It could also be worth trying a multi-vitamin/mineral supplement. There's some evidence that vitamin C reduces the tendency of sperm to stick together, making it easier for them to swim singly toward their target, and extra

vitamin E can lead to a significant improvement in sperm function, especially in the process whereby the sperm binds to the egg. (One study suggested this cheap and simple treatment could help up to one-fifth of men with sperm abnormalities.) Zinc also plays an important part in sperm production, while selenium can help sperm motility.

○ Removing a varicocele results in an improvement in semen quality for 50–75 per cent of men.

○ Men who suffer from blocked tubes, retrograde ejaculation, or erection problems can have their sperm collected surgically for artificial insemination. Artificial insemination, sometimes combined with 'sperm washing' (to remove poor quality sperm), can also be used in cases where sperm quantity and quality are low.

○ Drugs may be used to suppress immune system function in men whose sperm are being attacked by antibodies.

○ A hormonal supplement can be prescribed if natural testosterone levels are too low.

○ More sophisticated procedures include various methods of *in vitro* fertilization (essentially sperm are mixed with an egg in the laboratory) and a procedure called intracytoplasmic sperm injection (ICSI). This involves a single healthy sperm being isolated and then injected directly into an egg which is then transplanted into the woman. Because it requires just one sperm, ICSI can be used for men who have very low sperm counts or with irreversible vasectomies.

○ Don't worry about too much sex adversely affecting your semen profile. It seems abstaining from sex can *increase* semen volume and total sperm counts but also *decrease* the number of healthy sperm. Older sperm are simply less dynamic than their younger brothers. On balance, there are few advantages from abstaining for more than two or three days. Intriguingly, Israeli research suggests that men with low sperm counts, or insufficient numbers of motile sperm, could significantly increase their fertility potential by having intercourse every day, or even twice a day, when their partner is ovulating.

WHAT'S THE OUTLOOK?

○ It depends. Some causes of male infertility, such as a varicocele, can be relatively easily treated. Others, such as blocked tubes, may be harder to rectify.

○ Your ability to access good-quality fertility treatment will vary within and between countries, but in many areas it's available only at a high cost, effectively preventing many men from obtaining the treatment they need.

○ If your partner is fertile and your problem cannot be corrected, you may need to consider the option of 'donor insemination'. This involves your partner being artificially inseminated by sperm donated for fertility treatment by another man.

○ Your ability to tackle an infertility problem can depend on how well you're able to cope emotionally. It's common for men to feel anxious and depressed, to blame themselves for their partner's disappointment and to see themselves as less of a man. Many men also worry that their partner will abandon them in favor of another man with fully functioning testicles. It's important for men with these feelings to try to talk about them, certainly with their partners and perhaps also with a specialist fertility counselor. Although it may not feel like this at first, a fertility problem is a medical issue and not any sort of reflection on a man's sexuality, potency, or virility.

PENIS PROBLEMS

Sexual dysfunctions affecting the penis are dealt with elsewhere. For information on erection difficulties (impotence) see page 246, for premature ejaculation see page 251, and for retarded ejaculation see page 253.

Balanitis

WHAT ARE THE MAIN SYMPTOMS?
○ Redness, soreness, and itching on the glans (tip) of the penis.
○ If the foreskin is also inflamed, the problem is called balanoposthitis.

WHAT'S THE RISK?
○ Balanitis is very common among uncircumcised men of all ages (it's unusual among circumcised men).

WHAT CAUSES IT?
○ Balanitis is a medical term for the inflammation of the glans due to a variety of causes. It's definitely not a sexually transmitted infection, although it understandably worries men who think it might be.
○ Balanitis is basically skin damage which then becomes infected with candida (a yeast) or micro-organisms including trichomonads, streptococci, and anaerobes.

○ Skin damage can be the result of chemical irritation (this can include an allergy to soap, washing detergent, condom latex, or spermicides) or even normal sexual activity.

○ Poor genital hygiene, a tight foreskin, and diabetes.

HOW CAN I PREVENT IT?

○ Ensure that your foreskin can be retracted, and if it can't, consult your doctor.

○ Keep your penis clean, especially under the foreskin, and use a lubricant with sex to prevent skin damage.

○ If you sweat a lot, try putting a barrier cream (e.g. zinc and castor oil) around your glans.

WHAT ARE THE MAIN TREATMENTS?

○ Wash your penis with mild, unperfumed soaps or simply with warm, salted water.

○ Avoid sex until the skin has healed.

○ Depending on the cause, a doctor could prescribe antibiotics or hydrocortisone, anti-fungal, or steroid creams.

○ You could also try aloe vera gel, a herbal remedy, while a candida infection might be helped by eating more natural yoghurt.

○ Recurrent balanitis can make the foreskin scarred and inelastic, and you may then be referred to a specialist for circumcision.

WHAT'S THE OUTLOOK?

○ The condition often clears up naturally or with simple treatments.

Cancer of the penis

WHAT ARE THE MAIN SYMPTOMS?

○ An ulcer (which may give a smelly discharge), a warty growth, or a red velvety patch, usually located under the foreskin where the tip of the penis joins the shaft.

○ There may also be swollen, grape-sized lymph nodes under the skin fold at the top of the leg.

WHAT'S THE RISK?

○ Fortunately very low: in the UK and USA there's just one case per 100,000 men each year.

○ Almost all of those affected are over 60, and it hardly ever occurs among circumcised men.

WHAT CAUSES IT?
- ○ Not washing under the foreskin, either because of poor personal hygiene or because the foreskin is too tight to be retracted.
- ○ A viral infection of the penis, such as penile warts, can also be a risk factor.
- ○ Men who smoke are more likely to be affected.

HOW CAN I PREVENT IT?
- ○ Wash regularly under your foreskin, and if you can't retract it, see your doctor for advice.
- ○ If you develop penile warts get them treated as soon as possible.
- ○ Quit smoking.

WHAT ARE THE MAIN TREATMENTS?
- ○ Surgery to remove the cancer, radiotherapy, or chemotherapy.
- ○ If surgery is used, part of the penis will almost certainly be removed.

WHAT'S THE OUTLOOK?
- ○ In terms of survival, good. If the cancer is detected early, 90 per cent of cases are cured.
- ○ If the cancer has spread, however, the survival rate falls to about 30 per cent.

Penis size

WHAT ARE THE MAIN SYMPTOMS?
- ○ There's a medical condition known as 'micropenis' in which the erect penis can be less than half an inch in length. Most doctors regard an erect penis that is too short to have satisfactory intercourse (less than two inches) as a medical problem.
- ○ The main problem with penis size is actually psychological: despite having a penis of average length (between five inches and seven inches), many men convince themselves that theirs is far too small.

WHAT'S THE RISK?
- ○ The risk of having a micropenis is minute; the risk of believing that your penis is too small is significantly higher.
- ○ One survey of over 7000 American men found that most wanted a longer penis.

WHAT CAUSES IT?
- ○ A micropenis is caused by a hormonal problem before birth.

○ Penis-size anxiety is fueled by schoolboy banter and myths, seeing pornography showing men with unusually large organs, and insensitive comments by a sexual partner.

○ Men who feel insecure about their masculinity may convince themselves that their small penis (as they perceive it) is somehow responsible.

HOW CAN I PREVENT IT?

○ You can't develop a micropenis as you get older: what you've already got can't shrink significantly.

○ The best way to prevent penis-size anxiety is to try to feel positive about yourself generally and not to believe that your personal worth is any more related to the length of your penis than it is to the size of your big toe.

WHAT ARE THE MAIN TREATMENTS?

○ For men with a micropenis, cosmetic surgery may add about an inch in length.

○ For men with penis-size anxiety, it may help to:

   ➲ Measure your penis properly. When you've an erection, push it down until it's horizontal. Measure along the top from the base of the penis (that's the pubic bone, not the flab covering it) to the tip.

   ➲ Look at it side-on in a mirror. You shouldn't try to judge your organ simply by peering down at it; this perspective will inevitably make it look shorter.

   ➲ Lose some weight. Abdominal fat can conceal up to two inches of your penis.

○ Avoid vacuum pumps which claim to lengthen your penis. They don't work.

○ Sex experts always say that what really counts is what you do with whatever you've got. It's undeniable that some partners are excited by the idea of a larger penis, but that doesn't mean that they can't still enjoy sex with someone whose penis is smaller than average.

○ See a counselor.

○ Consider cosmetic surgery as an option. But it can have side-effects: your penis, when erect, will flop about rather than stand up; if you have fat added to increase your girth, it has a tendency to coalesce into unsightly lumps, and you may also need regular fat top-ups. (See page 222 for more information about the pros and cons of cosmetic surgery.)

WHAT'S THE OUTLOOK?

○ It depends very much on what you believe about your penis. If you have a surgically enhanced micropenis, it will probably still be shorter than average and you will have to find a way of coming to terms with that. If you are anxious about an already average-sized organ, you may need to make the effort to understand the underlying causes of your concern.

Peyronie's Disease

WHAT ARE THE MAIN SYMPTOMS?
○ Hard lumps which can be felt inside the shaft of the penis and/or a penis that bends when erect. The bend can be anywhere on the penis.
○ In some cases, the early stages of the disease are also painful.
○ The condition can make sexual activity difficult, if not impossible.

WHAT'S THE RISK?
○ Not great. One US study found about one in every 300 men were affected, although this is probably an under-estimate because some men are too embarrassed to see their doctor about it.
○ Although men of any age can develop this condition, the average age is around 50.

WHAT CAUSES IT?
○ Although finding a lump in the penis is understandably worrying, this condition isn't caused by cancer and isn't life-threatening.
○ Peyronie's Disease is caused by the presence of 'fibrous plaques' (scar tissue) within the penis. These have the same effect as sticking a piece of tape on one side of a long, thin balloon. When it's blown up, the tape prevents the area it covers from expanding properly, causing the inflated balloon to bend.
○ It may develop if damage has been caused by simply turning over awkwardly in bed with an erection during sleep. 'Missing the target' during penetration or vigorous sexual intercourse can also create problems.
○ Medical procedures that involve passing tubes or instruments through the urethra can increase the risk.

HOW CAN I PREVENT IT?
○ There's very little you can do, except perhaps be careful not to bend the penis too much during sex.

WHAT ARE THE MAIN TREATMENTS?
○ Some cases get better on their own so your doctor might advise 'waiting and watching' for a while.

○ A long-term vitamin E supplement or the drug Potaba can help some men.
○ Surgery is the last-resort solution for men who are unable to have pain-free sex. It's important to wait until the penis has stopped bending—if surgery is premature, the penis can continue to bend afterwards.

WHAT'S THE OUTLOOK?
○ Difficult to say, as Peyronie's Disease doesn't always follow a predictable course.

Phimosis

WHAT ARE THE MAIN SYMPTOMS?
○ A tightness of the foreskin which prevents it being drawn back over the glans.
○ A difficulty in urinating (causing the foreskin to balloon out).
○ Painful erections.
○ Problems with masturbation and sexual intercourse. The pain may cause a loss of erection during sex.
○ There is a related condition, called paraphimosis, which causes pain and swelling in the glans (the tip of the penis). In this condition, a tight foreskin retracts behind the glans and can't return to its normal position.

WHAT'S THE RISK?
○ A non-retractable foreskin is natural and common in infants—at birth only four per cent of foreskins are fully retractable—but by the age of 17, only one per cent of boys still have foreskins that aren't fully retractable.
○ There's a small risk of the problem starting during adulthood, mostly among older men.

WHAT CAUSES IT?
○ A naturally tight foreskin.
○ An infection or scarring (perhaps from an injury during sex).
○ Paraphimosis is usually caused by phimosis.

HOW CAN I PREVENT IT?
○ Keep yourself clean.

WHAT ARE THE MAIN TREATMENTS?
○ Some doctors will attempt plastic surgery to enlarge the foreskin, but this procedure doesn't often work.

○ Circumcision.

○ In early cases of paraphimosis, a doctor can often massage the foreskin back over the glans using an a ice-pack and lubricating gel. In persistent cases, circumcision may be necessary.

WHAT'S THE OUTLOOK?

○ Good, because effective treatments are available, although a circumcision will cause short-term discomfort and may reduce the sensitivity of the tip of the penis.

Priapism

WHAT ARE THE MAIN SYMPTOMS?

○ A prolonged and painful erection of the penis. Blood that has inflated the penis doesn't drain away after sexual stimulation has ended.

○ Normal erections last, on average, no longer than an hour among men in their early 20s and about 20 minutes for a man in his 50s or early 60s.

○ An erection that fails to subside after four hours is a medical emergency.

WHAT'S THE RISK?

○ Very small, although it's slightly greater for men with an underlying blood disorder (e.g. sickle-cell anemia) or who are using injection treatments for erectile dysfunction (impotence). The latest generation of injectable drugs is much less likely to cause this problem, however.

WHAT CAUSES IT?

○ A blood disorder.

○ Priapism following an injection treatment is caused by too high a dose of the drug.

○ The problem can also occur for no obvious reason.

HOW CAN I PREVENT IT?

○ You can't.

WHAT ARE THE MAIN TREATMENTS?

○ Two self-help treatments could be worth a try: a cold press (e.g. ice cubes wrapped in a towel) and exercise, either by running up and down stairs or using an exercise bicycle. But don't spend too much time on these if they don't work: if priapism isn't treated quickly, it can result in damage to the structure of the penis

and possibly impotence. Ignore your embarrassment and go straight to a doctor.
- O Draining off the blood with a syringe or administering drugs to shrink blood vessels and reduce inflow to the penis.
- O If it's caused by an injection treatment for erectile dysfunction, talk to your doctor about using a lower dose or a different treatment altogether.

WHAT'S THE OUTLOOK?
- O Good, if prompt treatment is sought.

PROSTATE PROBLEMS

The prostate gland is located beneath the bladder and is wrapped around the urethra, the tube that takes urine out through the penis. Its function is to produce fluids that keep sperm healthy, and it provides up to one-third of semen volume. Even though it's no larger than a walnut, the prostate can certainly cause some big problems.

Benign prostatic hyperplasia

This condition is also known as benign prostatic hypertrophy, and is usually abbreviated to BPH.

WHAT ARE THE MAIN SYMPTOMS?
- O Difficulty in starting to urinate.
- O A weak stream.
- O Starting and stopping in the middle of urinating.
- O Having to strain to urinate.
- O Discomfort when urinating.
- O Having to rush urgently to the toilet.
- O Having to urinate more often (including visiting the toilet more than once during the night).
- O A feeling of not having fully emptied the bladder.
- O A sudden inability to urinate.
- O Blood in the urine.

WHAT'S THE RISK?
- O High. BPH affects about one man in three over the age of 50. Younger men rarely develop the disease.

WHAT CAUSES IT?

O An enlargement of the prostate gland, causing it to constrict the urethra through which urine passes from the bladder to the penis. It's not caused by cancer, although the symptoms in the early stages are very similar to those of prostate cancer.
O One theory is that prostate cells may begin to grow as they become more sensitive to testosterone with ageing.
O A high-fat diet and obesity have been suggested as risk factors, but there's no conclusive proof.
O BPH can run in families.

HOW CAN I PREVENT IT?

O A low-fat diet and keeping your weight down might help. Soya products might also reduce your risk since they contain ingredients called phyto-estrogens which counteract the effects of testosterone.

WHAT ARE THE MAIN TREATMENTS?

O In mild cases, the doctor might recommend 'watching and waiting', i.e. taking no action unless the symptoms worsen.
O A zinc supplement may help reduce the size of the prostate and the severity of the symptoms.
O Alpha blockers, drugs which ease urinary problems by relaxing muscles in the prostate gland and the bladder neck.
O Finasteride, a so-called 5-Alpha-reductase inhibitor drug, which inhibits the action of testosterone on the prostate gland and causes it to shrink.
O There's increasing evidence that two herbal remedies—rye pollen extract and saw palmetto—can relieve BPH symptoms.
O Surgery. In more severe cases of BPH, the doctor may recommend a transurethral prostatectomy (TURP). An instrument is inserted down the penis to remove part of the enlarged prostate.

WHAT'S THE OUTLOOK?

O Many cases of BPH improve over time without any medical treatment.
O If the symptoms are intolerable, they can usually be controlled or relieved by drugs or surgery, although the price paid may be some unpleasant side-effects, such as incontinence, impotence, loss of libido, or retrograde ejaculation (where semen flows into the bladder rather than out of the penis).

TO SCREEN OR NOT TO SCREEN

It's now possible to be screened for early signs of prostate cancer before any obvious symptoms appear. The screening process involves a 'digital rectal' examination (in other words, the doctor feels your prostate with a finger inserted through the anus—this sounds worse than it is) and a blood test (for a substance called prostate-specific antigen or PSA). If these tests indicate a strong possibility of cancer, a sample of prostatic tissue will be removed for testing to get a definite result.

But doctors are divided as to whether a man without any symptoms should opt for screening. These are the main arguments:

The case for screening

○ In the USA, before screening became widespread, about one-third of men diagnosed with prostate cancer had advanced disease; now, with screening, only five per cent of all diagnosed men have advanced prostate cancer.
○ Cancers detected early can now be successfully treated. This virtually eliminates any worry about how fast the cancer might grow and spread.
○ Prostate checks can help doctors detect and treat other non-cancerous prostate problems. A digital rectal examination and the blood test for PSA can also indicate benign prostate enlargement (BPH) and prostatitis.

The case against screening

○ Prostate cancer is primarily a disease of old age, and many men with prostate cancer die of something else first anyway.
○ Since doctors have no way of knowing how fast a tumor will grow and spread, many men could end up having unnecessary treatment for what might have been a slow-growing cancer. (Only half of all cancers may actually be clinically significant.) What's more, surgery and radiotherapy can cause their own problems, including erectile dysfunction (impotence) and urinary incontinence.
○ Because the digital rectal examination and the blood test for PSA aren't very accurate, many men will be caused needless anxiety while they wait for a biopsy that turns out to show no signs of cancer. Only one-third of those with high PSA levels actually have cancer. A biopsy can itself cause health problems, including bleeding and infections.

TO SCREEN OR NOT TO SCREEN

Doctors in favor of prostate screening recommend that all men should have an annual test after the age of 50, although men at higher risk (because a relative developed the disease) should consider it annually from the age of 40. You best bet is to discuss the value of screening with your doctor.

Prostate cancer

WHAT ARE THE MAIN SYMPTOMS?
O They're the same as for benign prostatic hyperplasia (see page 240).

WHAT'S THE RISK?
O It's very common, especially in Europe, North America, and Australia. About 10 per cent of men develop the disease, although the symptoms are unlikely to appear in men aged under 60.
O About 40 per cent of men aged 80 have prostate cancer, although many of those cases are so mild they cause few if any symptoms.
O African-American men are at particularly high risk, perhaps as much as one-third higher than white men. Japanese and Chinese men are at much lower risk, however.
O If your father, brother, uncle, or grandfather has developed prostate cancer, you're at significantly greater risk. Men in families with a high incidence of breast cancer among women are also more likely to develop prostate cancer.
O The incidence of prostate cancer is increasing steadily. This is due in part to more cases being detected but there's also good evidence that more men are contracting the disease.

WHAT CAUSES IT?
O Scientists haven't yet pinpointed the cause, but a high-fat diet is a prime suspect. It could have an effect on key sex hormones, such as testosterone, that control cell growth within the prostate.

HOW CAN I PREVENT IT?
O Eat less fat, especially saturated fat.
O Eat more vegetables: vegetarians run half the risk of meat-eaters.

○ Tuck into tomatoes. Research suggests that the more tomato products you eat, the less likely you are to develop prostate cancer.
○ Quit smoking. This will increase your chances of surviving if you develop prostate cancer.

WHAT ARE THE MAIN TREATMENTS?
○ If the cancer is confined to the prostate there are three main options:
➲ 'Watchful waiting'. If your cancer appears to be developing slowly and isn't causing intolerable symptoms, some doctors will recommend taking no action apart from monitoring the problem. There's always the danger, however, that the cancer will start to spread more rapidly than expected.
➲ Surgery. Doctors are increasingly performing an operation known as a radical prostatectomy, the complete removal of the prostate gland. This is a major procedure, and although it is a very effective treatment, it often results in serious side-effects: up to 27 per cent of men become incontinent, and between 20 and 85 per cent suffer from erectile dysfunction (impotence).
➲ Radiotherapy. This is less invasive than surgery but may not eliminate the cancer entirely. It can also cause side-effects such as diarrhea or bleeding in the rectum, and between 40 and 67 per cent of men are affected by erectile dysfunction.
○ If the cancer is more advanced and has spread beyond the prostate gland, the options include radiotherapy and reducing testosterone levels through drugs or removing the testicles.

WHAT'S THE OUTLOOK?
○ If the cancer is identified before it's spread beyond the prostate, the chances of long-term survival are very good.
○ If the cancer has spread, however, average survival rates are reduced to just a few years.

Prostatitis

WHAT ARE THE MAIN SYMPTOMS?
○ Chills and fever.
○ Frequent urination.
○ Pain and difficulty in urinating.
○ Pain and discomfort in the prostate, scrotum, testes, penis, rectum, lower back,

lower abdomen, or inner thighs. There may also be pain between the scrotum and anus.
- A discharge from the penis.
- Pain on ejaculation.
- Blood in the semen.

WHAT'S THE RISK?
- High—at least one man in three suffers from a form of prostatitis at some stage. The peak age is 25–45.

WHAT CAUSES IT?
- There are three main types of prostatitis: acute and chronic bacterial prostatitis and chronic non-bacterial prostatitis. All these conditions are an inflammation of the prostate gland. There's also a related condition, known as prostatodynia, which produces similar symptoms but without any inflammation.
- Bacterial prostatitis can be caused by bacteria from the gut or sexually transmitted infections.
- Non-bacterial prostatitis and prostatodynia are less well understood. Possible causes include an increased stickiness of prostatic secretions or urine being forced into the prostate gland because of an abnormal emptying of the bladder.
- Prostatodynia has also been linked to stress.

HOW CAN I PREVENT IT?
- Practice safer sex to reduce the risk of infection.
- Have regular ejaculations to prevent fluid building up and congesting the gland.

WHAT ARE THE MAIN TREATMENTS?
- Antibiotics (if there is evidence of a bacterial infection) and pain killers (usually anti-inflammatories, e.g. ibuprofen).
- A new treatment for bacterial prostatitis, whose effectiveness has yet to be fully proven, is regular prostatic massage combined with antibiotics.
- Plenty of non-alcoholic, non-caffeinated fluids. Cranberry juice may help to relieve bacterial prostatitis.
- There's growing evidence that rye pollen extracts can relieve non-bacterial prostatitis and prostatodynia.
- There's anecdotal evidence that recovery can be speeded up by frequent ejaculations combined with Kegel exercises. These enable you to expel larger amounts of prostatic fluid in your semen (see page 178).

○ Prostatodynia can be treated by microwave warming of the prostate and drugs known as alpha blockers. Finding better ways of tackling stress could also help.

WHAT'S THE OUTLOOK?
○ With appropriate treatment, acute prostatitis can clear up within a week. Some cases may persist for several years, however, causing near-constant pain which is both debilitating and depressing. It'll help if you can find a doctor who understands the condition and takes it seriously.

SEXUAL DYSFUNCTIONS

Erectile dysfunction (impotence)

WHAT ARE THE MAIN SYMPTOMS?
○ The persistent inability to achieve or maintain an erection good enough to complete your chosen sexual activity satisfactorily, whether that's masturbation, oral sex, or vaginal or anal intercourse.

WHAT'S THE RISK?
○ It's a virtual certainty that every man will be unable to get an erection at least once in his lifetime. This could be due to stress, exhaustion, too much alcohol, or simply not feeling like sex.
○ Longer-term erection problems are estimated to affect about 10 per cent of men at any one time.
○ Although age itself isn't a cause of erectile dysfunction (ED), the risk nevertheless increases as you get older: those aged 50–59 are over three-and-a-half times more likely to be affected than those aged 18–29, and while 40 per cent of men are impotent at 40, the proportion rises to 67 per cent by the age of 70.

WHAT CAUSES IT?
○ There are two main causes of ED: physiological and psychological. Most doctors agree that the majority of cases are physiological, although there is disagreement about the exact proportions. It's clear, however, that even if a man's ED has primarily physical causes, he's soon likely to feel anxious, stressed, or depressed, psychological states that could well reinforce his physical problem.

○ The main physical causes are:
➲ Diabetes. Up to 25 per cent of all diabetic men aged 30–34 are affected by ED, as are 75 per cent of men aged 60–64.
➲ Inadequate blood flow to the penis because arteries have become furred-up or damaged. This causes about 40 per cent of ED cases in men aged over 50. Excessive drainage of blood from the penis can also cause ED.
➲ The side-effect of prescribed drugs, particularly those used to treat high blood pressure, heart disease, depression, peptic ulcers, and cancer. As many as 25 per cent of ED cases may be caused by drugs taken to treat other conditions.
➲ Spinal-cord injury.
➲ Smoking.
➲ Excessive drinking.
➲ Prostate-gland surgery (or other surgery around the pelvis).
➲ Hormonal imbalances.
○ The main psychological causes are:
➲ Relationship conflicts.
➲ Stress and anxiety.
➲ Depression.
➲ Unresolved sexual orientation.
➲ Sexual boredom.
○ One rough-and-ready way of working out whether your ED has a physical cause is to see whether there any circumstances in which you get an erection. If you can produce one when masturbating but not with a partner, wake up with an erection, or have erections during the night, then there's a good chance that your ED has psychological causes.

HOW CAN I PREVENT IT?
○ Have a healthy lifestyle. A low-fat diet, regular aerobic exercise, quitting smoking, drinking alcohol in moderation, and coping better with stress will all help.
○ If you have diabetes, ensure it's properly controlled.

WHAT ARE THE MAIN TREATMENTS?
○ *Oral drugs.* The first, and best known, oral treatment is Viagra (the name for sildenafil). It works by helping to relax the blood vessels in the penis, allowing blood to flow in. It doesn't work unless you're also sexually stimulated. The most common side-effects are headaches and facial flushing, and it can't be taken by men who are also using medicines containing nitrates (commonly

RIDING LOW

Cycling's great for your general health but could cause some surprising problems for your sex life: it's recently been recognized as a cause of erectile dysfunction. The most common problem is simply falling onto the crossbar—at 20 mph this puts a quarter of a ton of force on the key blood vessel and nerves running to the penis. But it seems that regular cycling could, over time, have a similar effect.

○ Doctors have measured a 66 per cent average reduction in blood flow through the artery running to the penis when cyclists are on a thin saddle and a 25 per cent reduction on a wide saddle.

○ It's been calculated that it takes only 11 per cent of a man's weight to compress the artery and frequent pressure of this sort could permanently affect its shape and performance.

○ A study of participants in a Norwegian bicycle touring race of 540 kilometers found that 20 per cent later experienced penile numbness; 13 per cent also reported ED—it lasted for more than one week for seven per cent of the participants and for more than one month for two per cent.

○ Regular club cyclists are much more likely to have ED problems than a comparable group of long-distance swimmers, according to a German study. It found that the likelihood of genital numbness among cyclists is directly related to the distances covered in training.

○ If you're a regular cyclist and suffer from ED, don't forget to mention this possible connection to your doctor. Protect yourself, too, by padding the cycle's crossbar and investing in a wider saddle. You can also stand up in the pedals every 10 minutes or so to keep the blood flowing.

prescribed for angina). Viagra shouldn't be used by men taking poppers (amyl nitrite) either, since these also contains nitrates. Other oral treatments are now beginning to become available; in some cases, these can be used by men for whom Viagra is not suitable.

○ *Injection therapy.* A tried-and-tested and reliable method of producing erections. You inject a drug, usually alprostadil, directly into the penis. This relaxes the blood vessels and muscles, allowing increased blood flow and producing an erection within 10–15 minutes. The main problems are that some men, understandably, don't like sticking a needle into their penis, there can be pain after the injection, and a few men develop nodules in the shaft. If the dose is too high, a prolonged erection can also occur (see the section on priapism, page 239).

WHAT MAKES MY PENIS GO UP?

Erections occur in a far from obvious way. Your penis is actually more active when it's limp than when it's erect. Seriously. When it's in this state, small muscles in your penis are tightly contracted to prevent blood flowing in. It's only when you're sexually aroused that these muscles relax, allowing blood to fill the spongy tissues that run the length of your penis. The blood can't flow straight out again because, as they enlarge, the spongy tissues press against the tough coating beneath the skin of the penis. This compresses small veins running just beneath the coating, stopping blood draining out of the penis. Your erection will fade away when the muscles in the arteries that bring blood into the penis contract, reducing the pressure on the small veins.

○ *MUSE (medicated urethral system for erection).* This method also uses alprostadil, but this time it's administered by means of a small pellet inserted into the urethra via a plastic applicator. It's less effective than injections, working for about two-thirds of men. The most common side-effect is penile pain, and partners may experience some burning if the drug leaks out during intercourse.

○ *Vacuum pumps.* You place your penis in a clear plastic cylinder and pump out the air, creating a vacuum. The penis becomes engorged with blood and, when it's firm enough, you place a plastic constricting ring around the base of the penis to trap the blood. There are few side-effects (apart from the occasional slight bruising), and the devices work for more than 90 per cent of men.

○ *Hormonal supplements.* Testosterone will be given to men in the relatively few cases where low levels are the cause of ED, especially if they also have low sexual desire.

○ *Penile implants.* A mechanical device is surgically inserted into the penis. It can be either permanently rigid or have a hydraulic action, operated via a valve in the scrotum. Although usually effective, implants are very much a last-ditch option and are less widely used now that so many other effective treatments are available.

○ *Sex therapy.* Whatever the cause or treatment of their ED, many men could benefit from counseling or therapy. In fact, the best treatment centers provide it as a matter of course. Sex therapy will be particularly necessary if the ED has psychological causes which can't actually be 'cured' with physical treatments. If a man has ED as a result of emotional conflict with a partner, for example, providing him with a drug that produces an erection isn't going to resolve that conflict; in fact, it might even make it worse. Men with physically caused ED may also have

WHAT CAN I DO ABOUT MY ERECTION PROBLEMS?

○ Get help and advice as soon as you notice a problem. This isn't important only in terms of getting treatment for your ED: it could also be a symptom of other potentially serious conditions (e.g. diabetes or heart disease).

○ If your doctor doesn't take your problem seriously, ask to be referred to a specialist. Don't let yourself be fobbed off with comments like 'What do you expect at your age?'

○ If you're prescribed a treatment that doesn't suit you, ask if you can try another. A wide variety are now available.

○ Don't try to treat yourself by seeking out pornography or asking a partner to wear erotic clothing or act out your fantasies. This almost certainly won't work and could leave you feeling even more upset.

○ Don't be tempted to buy herbal supplements or so-called aphrodisiacs through the Internet or magazine advertisements. You can't be sure what you're getting and these remedies are very unlikely to work.

○ Share your worries. No, you don't have to tell people you meet at the bus stop about your penis problems, but it will help enormously if you can talk to someone you trust. It's particularly important to communicate with your partner. Some men try to deal with their ED by hiding it from their partner and make all sorts of excuses for not attempting sex. This can cause feelings of confusion and rejection as well as suspicions that you're having an affair. You best bet is to be as open and honest as possible with your partner and ask for support.

○ Place less emphasis on intercourse and more on developing other forms of sexual intimacy. Spending time cuddling, kissing, licking, and massaging can still be pleasurable and will help keep you emotionally close to your partner.

○ Don't blame yourself for your ED. It's a health problem and not a reflection of your masculinity. Don't be tempted to blame your partner either.

lost a great deal of self-esteem and sexual confidence which sex therapy could help restore. It usually makes sense also to involve any permanent partner in sex therapy since the restoration, as well as the loss, of a man's erectile functioning will almost inevitably profoundly affect their relationship.

WHAT'S THE OUTLOOK?

○ There's an excellent chance that your erections can be restored but the psychological scars may take longer, and be harder, to heal.

Loss of sexual desire

WHAT ARE THE MAIN SYMPTOMS?
○ You don't feel like having sex.

WHAT'S THE RISK?
○ Surprisingly high—about 15 per cent of men aged 18–59 say they lack interest in sex, according to a recent large survey.

WHAT CAUSES IT?
○ There are a wide range of causes, including relationship difficulties, sexual boredom, depression, exhaustion, stress, and a low level of testosterone.
○ It's possible that you simply have a naturally lower level of sexual desire than your partner and that your real problem is finding a way to negotiate some sort of compromise.

HOW CAN I PREVENT IT?
○ Improve the quality of your sleep, cope better with stress, sort out any relationship problems, find ways of spicing up your sex life.
○ Get help if you're depressed.
○ Regular exercise may also increase your sense of well-being and feelings of sexual desire.

WHAT ARE THE MAIN TREATMENTS?
○ Sex therapy and, in a few cases, testosterone supplements.
○ Talk to your partner about your feelings and find ways of developing intimacy and closeness that aren't linked only to sex.
○ Avoid quack remedies, including so-called aphrodisiacs—there's no good evidence that any of them work.

WHAT'S THE OUTLOOK?
○ Good.

Premature (or rapid) ejaculation

WHAT ARE THE MAIN SYMPTOMS?
○ Ejaculation that occurs more quickly than a man and his partner would wish, causing problems in a sexual relationship.

○ The usual problem is that a man will come during penetration itself or very soon afterwards.

WHAT'S THE RISK?
○ It's a very common problem—in fact, it's the most common sexual dysfunction affecting men.
○ About one in three men of all ages suffers from premature ejaculation.

WHAT CAUSES IT?
○ It's very rarely caused by a physical problem.
○ The most common causes include stress, anxiety about sex (perhaps because of a fear of pregnancy, of a sexually transmitted infection, or of failing to perform adequately), relationship difficulties, and the lasting effects of teenage sexual experiences that had to be quick to avoid detection.

HOW CAN I PREVENT IT?
○ There's not much you can do, except find better ways of coping with stress and resolving difficulties with your partner.

WHAT ARE THE MAIN TREATMENTS?
○ You could try these short-term remedies (although they won't necessarily tackle the underlying problem):
  ➲ Increase the frequency of ejaculations, perhaps by masturbation. This could have the effect of delaying subsequent ejaculations.
  ➲ Wear a condom, or use an anesthetic spray, to reduce the sensitivity of your penis.
  ➲ Don't focus on penetration during sex. You may be able to ease the pressure on yourself if you don't attempt penetration until your partner has already had an orgasm.
○ Sex therapy. This is normally based on two techniques:
  ➲ *Stop-start.* You stimulate your penis (or ask your partner to do it for you) until you're near the point of ejaculation. Then stop and rest for 30–60 seconds before stimulating your penis again. You repeat this process five or six times in each 'training' session.
  ➲ *Squeeze.* You stimulate your penis (or ask your partner to do it for you) until you're near the point of ejaculation. This time, you firmly squeeze the tip of your penis: put your thumb on the underside of the penis in the indent where the head meets the shaft (the frenulum) and your first and second

fingers on the other side of the penis, just above and below the ridge that separates the head from the shaft. The squeeze has the effect of preventing ejaculation.

The idea of both these techniques is that, over time, you'll start to recognize what it feels like to near the moment when you can't stop yourself coming. When you're able to do that during sex itself, you can then take steps to slow down or stop whatever you're doing until the feeling fades. Once you know you can control your ejaculation in this way, your confidence increases, and eventually the whole process becomes unconscious and automatic.

○ Drugs. In some cases, doctors will prescribe particular anti-depressant drugs that, as a side-effect, slow down your body's progress toward ejaculation. The problems with this treatment are that you end up taking powerful medication designed to treat a completely different condition and the drugs don't always work anyway.

WHAT'S THE OUTLOOK?
○ With determination and persistence, it's possible to develop ejaculatory control.

Retarded ejaculation

WHAT ARE THE MAIN SYMPTOMS?
○ The inability to ejaculate or a long delay before ejaculation.

WHAT'S THE RISK?
○ About one man in 20 is affected.

WHAT CAUSES IT?
○ Most of the causes are psychological, including performance anxiety, self-consciousness, a belief that sex is somehow dirty or immoral, stress, and relationship difficulties.
○ It can also be the result of nerve damage or a side-effect of certain anti-depressant drugs.

HOW CAN I PREVENT IT?
○ There's not much you can do, except find better ways of coping with stress, and resolving difficulties with your partner.

WHAT ARE THE MAIN TREATMENTS?
○ Relaxation exercises, 'superstimulation' (e.g. using a vibrator or body oil combined with vigorous rubbing), sex therapy, or a large dose of a drug called yohimbine.
○ Avoid penetration until you're very near the point of ejaculation.
○ It may be necessary to change any drugs that might be causing the problem.

WHAT'S THE OUTLOOK?
○ Good, with determination and persistence.

TESTICLE PROBLEMS

Epididymitis

WHAT ARE THE MAIN SYMPTOMS?
○ Severe pain in the scrotum; swelling that may feel hot to the touch; fever.

WHAT'S THE RISK?
○ Low.

WHAT CAUSES IT?
○ Bacteria infect the epididymis, the tube leading from the testicle to the vas deferens. Chlamydia or gonorrhea can sometimes be responsible.

HOW CAN I PREVENT IT?
○ Practice safer sex (always use a condom during intercourse) and have regular check-ups for sexually transmitted infections.

WHAT ARE THE MAIN TREATMENTS?
○ Antibiotics. Also rest, take pain killers, and apply an ice-pack to your scrotum.

WHAT'S THE OUTLOOK?
○ Good, although in some cases the scrotum will remain abnormally enlarged.

Hydrocele

WHAT ARE THE MAIN SYMPTOMS?
○ Soft and usually painless swelling of the scrotum. In extreme cases, it can grow to the size of a grapefruit.

WHAT'S THE RISK?
- Low.

WHAT CAUSES IT?
- A build-up of fluid in the scrotum, sometimes caused by an injury to the testicles.

HOW CAN I PREVENT IT?
- Not much can be done, except to protect the testicles during sport.

WHAT ARE THE MAIN TREATMENTS?
- Usually none, unless the swelling has become large and uncomfortable. Large hydroceles can be drained through a syringe; more commonly, surgery is used to remove excess tissue from the sac containing the hydrocele.

WHAT'S THE OUTLOOK?
- Most cases can be permanently treated.

Testicular cancer

WHAT ARE THE MAIN SYMPTOMS?
- A swelling or lump in either testicle.
- A 'heavy' feeling in the testicle.
- Sometimes a dull ache and, rarely, acute pain in the scrotum.

WHAT'S THE RISK?
- It's relatively rare: the risk of the disease is about one in 450 over a lifetime, and it mainly affects men aged 15–35.
- Men born with undescended testicles are at five times greater risk.
- The brother of a man with testicular cancer has a nine times greater chance of developing the disease than average, and sons of fathers who have developed the condition are at four times greater risk.
- Testicular cancer is becoming more common: the incidence has doubled over the past 20 years in many countries.

WHAT CAUSES IT?
- It's not entirely clear, although there's clearly a strong genetic element. It's also been linked to environmental pollutants (e.g. DDT, other pesticides, and PCBs)

REAL HEALTH FOR MEN

GETTING ON THE BALLS

All men should check their testicles regularly for signs of cancer.
Here's how to do it:

○ The best time is after a bath or shower when the muscle in the scrotal sac
  is more relaxed.
○ Hold your scrotum in the palms of both hands.
○ Note the size and weight of the testicles. It's usual to have one slightly
  larger testicle or for one to hang lower than the other. Watch out for any
  noticeable increase in size or weight.
○ Still supporting your scrotum, use the fingers and thumbs on both hands to
  feel each testicle in turn. You should be able to feel a soft tube at the top
  and back of the testicle. This is the epididymis which carries and stores
  sperm. You should also be able to feel the smooth, firm tube of the
  spermatic cord which runs up from the epididymis.
○ Each testicle should feel smooth with no lumps or swellings.
○ If you do notice any changes, see your doctor as soon as possible. Most
  testicular lumps are non-cancerous, but a few will need further investigation.
○ It's especially important to check your testicles regularly if you were born
  with undescended testicles or if a close relative has had the disease.

---

which could effect the development of male fetuses while still in the womb.
○ Men with a sedentary lifestyle may be at greater risk, but this hasn't been
  proved conclusively.

HOW CAN I PREVENT IT?
○ You can't.

WHAT ARE THE MAIN TREATMENTS?
○ There's currently no option but to remove the affected testicle, although
  alternative treatments are being investigated.
○ Chemotherapy or radiotherapy are often used as supplementary treatments to
  surgery.

WHAT'S THE OUTLOOK?
○ Generally good. Testicular cancer is one of the easiest cancers to treat, with

cure rates exceeding 95 per cent in cases that are detected early, and the removal of one testicle doesn't normally have any long-term affects on fertility or sexual performance. But survival rates are lower if the cancer has had time to spread, making it essential that you see a doctor as soon as you become aware of a possible problem.

○ Perhaps surprisingly, most men deal very well with the psychological consequences of losing a testicle because of cancer. Very few feel 'less of a man' as a result.

Torsion

WHAT ARE THE MAIN SYMPTOMS?
○ Sudden, severe pain in a testicle, often combined with abdominal pain and fever.

WHAT'S THE RISK?
○ Low. It's most common in teenage boys and rare after the mid 20s.

WHAT CAUSES IT?
○ The spermatic cord that supports the testicles becomes twisted, cutting off the blood supply. It's not known why it happens, but it's more common among men with unusually mobile testicles.

HOW CAN I PREVENT IT?
○ You can't.

WHAT ARE THE MAIN TREATMENTS?
○ It's a medical emergency requiring surgery. It's vital to see a doctor within four hours to prevent irreversible damage to the testicle.

WHAT'S THE OUTLOOK?
○ Good, if treatment is carried out quickly. If left untreated for too long, the affected testicle may have to be removed.

Varicocele

WHAT ARE THE MAIN SYMPTOMS?
○ A usually painless swelling, commonly on the left testicle. It's often more prominent when you stand up. There may also be a 'dragging' feeling.

WHAT'S THE RISK?

○ 10–15 per cent of men develop a varicocele.

WHAT CAUSES IT?

○ A collection of varicose veins within the scrotum.

HOW CAN I PREVENT IT?

○ You can't.

WHAT ARE THE MAIN TREATMENTS?

○ A technique known as embolization. This involves inserting small tungsten coils to block the veins leading to the varicocele.

WHAT'S THE OUTLOOK?

○ Good, but varicoceles can recur.

Testosterone deficiency

This condition is known medically as hypogonadism.

WHAT ARE THE MAIN SYMPTOMS?

○ A reduction in facial hair growth.
○ Loss of body hair.
○ Shrinking testicles.
○ Loss of sex drive.
○ Erectile dysfunction (impotence).
○ Infertility.
○ A loss of muscle bulk and increasing muscle weakness.
○ Tiredness and depression.

WHAT'S THE RISK?

○ It's rare, affecting about five men in every thousand.

WHAT CAUSES IT?

○ A genetic defect called Klinefelter's Syndrome.
○ The surgical removal of both testicles (after an accident, for example).
○ A disease of the hypothalamus or pituitary gland.
○ Testicular failure for no obvious cause.

WHAT ABOUT THE MALE MENOPAUSE?

If you're between 35 and 60 do any of these symptoms seem familiar?

○ A loss of interest in sex and less powerful erections.

○ A loss of drive at work.

○ Feelings of fatigue, lethargy, exhaustion, or depression.

○ A sense of hopelessness and helplessness.

○ Stiff or painful joints or muscles.

○ Irritability.

○ Hot flushes/flashes.

If so, you could be experiencing the so-called 'male menopause' (also dubbed the 'andropause' or 'viropause'), at least according to some doctors. Their argument is that as men get older these symptoms are caused by falling levels of 'bio-available' testosterone (although testosterone levels do not fall enough to cause hypogonadism). This happens not only because testosterone production declines during and after middle age but also because levels of another hormone (SHBG, sex-hormone-binding globulin) rise. SHBG has the effect of reducing the levels of active testosterone in the blood. Normal levels of active testosterone can be restored by hormone replacement therapy, a treatment that effectively rejuvenates flagging middle-aged men.

Most doctors believe the scientific evidence for the male menopause is weak, however. Men's testosterone levels do fall after the age of 25, but only by a gradual one per cent a year. There's also no evidence for a dramatic change in SHBG levels. Testosterone replacement therapy can't tackle erectile dysfunction (except for the few men who do have seriously low testosterone levels), and its advocates haven't yet proved scientifically that it relieves any of the other physical and emotional problems typically experienced by middle-aged men. There's also a worry that testosterone supplements could stimulate prostate enlargement, both benign and cancerous.

It's much more likely that many of the male menopause symptoms are actually either stress-related or connected to the emotional trauma of passing through middle age. This means that they require much more than a simple drug treatment. See pages 125–6 for suggestions about how middle-aged men can start to come to terms with what can certainly be a confusing period of change and uncertainty.

WHAT IS TESTOSTERONE?

It's the key male hormone; in fact, it's what makes us male. Without it, a fetus won't develop male characteristics. In infancy, testosterone makes sure our testicles descend, and in puberty it stimulates body hair, voice deepening, muscle development, and sex drive. Our testicles normally produce 3–10 mg of testosterone a day, although the level is higher in the morning than at night. If you want to boost your levels naturally, avoid too much booze and cannabis, start a regular exercise program and have lots of sex (especially hours of foreplay—no kidding, all that excitement's great for your hormones as well as making your semen more fertile).

HOW CAN I PREVENT IT?
○ You can't.

WHAT ARE THE MAIN TREATMENTS?
○ Testosterone replacement therapy. This can be supplied via a skin patch, injection, an implant under the skin, or tablets taken orally.
○ Avoid any non-medical herbal remedies (e.g. wild yam) for boosting your testosterone levels. Even if any of them do increase your testosterone production, the effect will be marginal and you'll have wasted your money.

WHAT'S THE OUTLOOK?
○ Good.

LIVE LONG AND PROSPER

Whether you've read some or all of this book, you'll have discovered information that could improve the quality of your life now as well as in the next 10, 20, or even 50 years. By making small but important changes to your lifestyle, you can not only feel better, have higher energy levels, and enjoy more satisfying sex but also add years to your lifespan.

If there's one key message running through this book, it's this: if you want to improve your health, start by thinking about yourself as a man. Men's health is generally much worse than it need be because we've been brought up to treat our bodies as if they're virtually indestructible. If we do develop a problem, we're likely to ignore it in the hope that it'll go away, and we tend not to ask for help until we're convinced it's really serious (by which time it probably is). This isn't an effective strategy for maintaining good health. We need to develop a more realistic view of our physical and emotional selves—one that reflects our vulnerabilities as well as our strengths—and accept that seeing a doctor isn't a sign of weakness or failure. Fortunately, there are many signs that many men's attitudes and behaviors are now changing, making it easier for more of us to feel comfortable about taking our health much more seriously.

The other big idea in this book is that health cannot easily be divided up into neat compartments. We can't become healthy simply by improving our diet or quitting smoking (although both these steps would help enormously). How well we deal with stress and the quality of our emotional lives and relationships with others can also make a huge difference. To be truly healthy, we need to understand that our body and mind are closely linked; in fact, some scientists argue that they're so intertwined that it's increasingly difficult to see them as distinct. Again, there are good indications that many men are now realizing that this 'holistic' view of health is not some namby-pamby New Age fad but actually offers a scientifically proven route to well-being.

If you want to give your health a major boost, you can't do much better than to make as many as possible of these 12 key changes:

○ **Get physically active.** Exercise can improve mood, strengthen bones, and reduce the risk of diabetes, heart disease, and cancer. It's never too late to start, and even regular brisk walking can make a big difference.

○ **Stop smoking.** It's a tough habit to kick, but the health improvements begin within just 20 minutes of your last cigarette. The obvious benefits aside, quitting makes erections firmer and increases sperm concentrations.

○ **Drink alcohol in moderation.** Sticking to one or two drinks a day will do much more than abolish hangovers: men aged over 40 who drink at this level have a lower risk of heart disease than men who drink excessively or who never drink at all.

○ **Eat more fruit and vegetables.** If you make only one change to your diet, do this. It'll cut your chances of developing heart disease and cancer—and should also come as a great relief to your hemorrhoids.

○ **Watch your weight.** Keeping your waist circumference below 37 inches will be good news not only for the seams on your trousers: it'll also reduce the risk of a premature death—and make your penis look longer.

○ **Express your emotions.** There are no longer any prizes for being the strong and silent type; in fact, becoming more aware of your emotions benefits your immune system and your heart.

○ **Value relationships.** Being part a rich social network boosts immune functioning and reduces the risks of heart disease and premature death. Even a relationship with a pet is good for your blood pressure.

○ **Enjoy a healthy sex life.** Becoming clearer about your sexual needs, knowing how to have safer sex, and being willing to tackle sexual problems will increase satisfaction between the sheets. Regular sex can also help keep you fit and even looking younger.

○ **Get a good night's sleep.** Sleep might seem boring but it's good for your immune system and mental health. If you're well-rested you'll not only feel and perform better but you might also live longer.

○ **Keep the lid on stress.** Effective stressbusting will not only make you feel better, it'll also improve your relationships, make work more satisfying, and reduce your risk of developing a wide range of diseases. Your testosterone levels could also rise—and your sex drive with it.

○ **Monitor your health.** The sooner any health problem is diagnosed the easier it is to tackle it. That means it's worth checking your testicles for lumps once a month and having your blood pressure measured at least once every three years.

○ **If you're worried about your health, get medical advice.** Your doctor won't think you're wasting his or her time, and the earlier you're treated the better your chances of a quick recovery.

Whatever your age and current level of health and fitness, there's no longer any doubt that you can significantly improve your health and well-being. You might not be able to change your whole lifestyle overnight (and it probably wouldn't be sensible to try), but you certainly no longer have to settle for just 'getting by,' 'doing okay,' or being 'all right.' Your goal can now be nothing less than Real Health.

APPENDIX

GETTING THE HELP YOU NEED

Organizations

Symbols
✉ Postal address
☎ Telephone
🖳 Website

UNITED KINGDOM

British Association for Counselling and Psychotherapy
✉ 1 Regent Place, Rugby, CV21 2PJ
☎ 01788 578328
🖳 www.bac.co.uk

British Heart Foundation
✉ 14 Fitzhardinge Street, London, W1H 6DH
☎ 020 7935 0185
🖳 www.bhf.org.uk

Drinkline
(for advice and information on reducing alcohol consumption)
☎ 0800 917 8282

Family Planning Association
(for advice and information on contraception, sexually transmitted infections, and other sexual health issues)
✉ 2–12 Pentonville Road, London, N1 9FP
☎ 0845 310 1334
🖳 www.fpa.org.uk

Fathers Direct
(for information, advice, and support for fathers)
✉ Herald House, Lambs Passage, Bunhill Row, London, EC1Y 8TQ
☎ 020 7920 9491
🖳 www.fathersdirect.com

Impotence Association
(for information and advice on all sexual dysfunctions)
✉ PO Box 10296, London, SW17 9WH
☎ 020 8767 7791
🖳 www.impotence.org.uk

Institute of Cancer Research
✉ 123 Old Brompton Road, London, SW7 3RP
☎ 020 7352 8133
🖥 www.icr.ac.uk

Imperial Cancer Research Fund
✉ 61 Lincoln's Inn Fields, London, WC2A 3PX
☎ 020 7242 0200
🖥 www.icnet.uk

ISSUE: The National Fertility Association
✉ 114 Lichfield Street, Walsall, West Midlands, WS1 1SZ
☎ 01922 722888
🖥 www.issue.co.uk

malehealth.co.uk
(A comprehensive men's health website)
🖥 www.malehealth.co.uk

Men's Health Helpline
(a telephone advice service for any male health problem)
☎ 020 8995 4448

National AIDS Helpline
☎ 0800 567123

The Orchid Cancer Appeal
(for information about prostate and testicular cancers)
✉ St Bartholomew's Hospital, London, EC1A 7BE
☎ 020 7601 7808
🖥 www.orchid-cancer.org.uk

The Prostate Cancer Charity
✉ 3 Angel Walk, London, W6 9HX
☎ 0845 300 8383
🖥 www.prostate-cancer.org.uk

Prostate Help Association
✉ Langworth, Lincoln, LN3 5DF
🖥 www.pha.u-net.com

Quitline
(for advice and information on stopping smoking)
☎ 0800 002200

Relate
(for counseling for relationship and/or sexual problems)
✉ Herbert Gray College, Little Church Street, Rugby, CV21 3AP
☎ 01788 573241
🖥 www.relate.org.uk

The Samaritans
(for emotional support for people in crisis or at risk of suicide)
☎ 08457 90 90 90
🖥 www.samaritans.org

The Terrence Higgins Trust
(for advice and information on HIV and Aids)
✉ 52–54 Grays Inn Road, London, WC1X 8JU
☎ 020 7242 1010
🖥 www.tht.org.uk

UNITED STATES OF AMERICA

American Foundation for Urologic Disease
(for prostate and testicular problems and sexual dysfunctions)
✉ 1128 North Charles Street, Baltimore, Maryland 21201
☎ 410-468-1800
🖥 www.afud.org

American Heart Association
✉ 7272 Greenville Avenue, Dallas, Texas 75231
☎ 1-800-AHA-USA1
🖥 www.americanheart.org

American Institute for Cancer Research
⊠ 1759 R Street NW, Washington, DC 20009
☎ 1-800-843-8114
🖳 www.aicr.org

American Institute of Stress
⊠ 124 Park Avenue, Yonkers, New York 10703
☎ 914-963-1200
🖳 www.stress.org

Cancer Information Service
☎ 1-800-422-6237
🖳 rex.nci.nih.gov

CDC National HIV and AIDS Hotline
⊠ PO Box 13827, Research Triangle Park, North Carolina 27709
☎ 1-800-342-2437
🖳 www.ashastd.org

CDC National STD Hotline
(for advice and information on sexually transmitted infections)
⊠ PO Box 13827, Research Triangle Park, North Carolina 27709
☎ 1-800-227-8922
🖳 www.ashastd.org

The Men's Health Network
⊠ PO Box 75972, Washington, DC 20013
☎ 202-543-MHN-1 (6461)
🖳 www.menshealthnetwork.org

National Depressive and Manic-Depressive Association
⊠ 730 N Franklin Street, Suite 501, Chicago, Illinois 60610-7204
☎ 800-826-3632
🖳 ndmda.org

National Mental Health Association
⊠ 1021 Prince Street, Alexandria, Virginia 22314-2971
☎ 703-684-7722
🖳 www.nmha.org

Prostate Action Inc.
⊠ PO Box 630947, Houston, Texas 77263-0947
☎ 713-785-3368
🖳 www.prostateaction.org

The Prostatitis Foundation
⊠ 1063 30th Street Box 8, Smithshire, Illinois 61478
☎ 1-888-891-4200
🖳 www.prostatitis.org

AUSTRALIA

ACCESS: Australia Infertility Network
⊠ PO Box 959, Parramatta, NSW 2124
☎ 02 9670 2380
🖳 www.access.org.au

The Australian Cancer Society
⊠ Level 4, 70 William Street, East Sydney, NSW 2011
☎ 02 9380 9022
🖳 www.cancer.org.au

Australian Federation of AIDS Organisations
⊠ Level 4, 74-78 Wentworth Avenue, Surry Hills, NSW 1300
☎ 02 9281 1999
🖳 www.afao.org.au

National Heart Foundation of Australia
⊠ Cnr Denison St & Geils Court, Deakin, ACT 2600
☎ 1300 36 27 87
🖳 www.heartfoundation.com.au

The National Tobacco Campaign
☎ 131 848
🖥 www.quitnow.info.au

Relationships Australia
(for relationship problems)
✉ PO Box 313, Curtin, ACT 2605.
☎ 02 6285 4466
🖥 www.relationships.com.au

SANE Australia
(for information and advice on depression, suicide, and other mental-health issues)
✉ PO Box 226, South Melbourne 3205
☎ 03 9682 5944
🖥 www.sane.org

NEW ZEALAND

Alcohol Drug Association New Zealand
✉ PO Box 13-496 Christchurch
☎ 03 379 8626
🖥 www.adanz.org.nz

Cancer Society of New Zealand
✉ PO Box 12-145, Wellington
☎ 04 494 7270
🖥 www.cancernz.org.nz

Mental Health Foundation
✉ PO Box 10051, Dominion Road, Auckland
☎ 09 630 8573
🖥 www.mentalhealth.org.nz

National Heart Foundation of New Zealand
✉ PO Box 17160, Greenlane, Auckland
☎ 09 571 9191

New Zealand AIDS Foundation
✉ PO Box 6663, Wellesley Street, Auckland
☎ 09 303 3124
🖥 www.nzaf.org.nz

CANADA

Canadian AIDS Society
✉ 4th Floor, 309 rue Cooper Street, Ottawa K2P 0G5
☎ 613 230 3580
🖥 www.cdnaids.ca

Canadian Cancer Society
✉ 10 Alcorn Avenue, Suite 200, Toronto, Ontario, M4V 3B1
☎ 1-888-939-3333
🖥 www.cancer.ca

Canadian Chronic Prostatitis Research Foundation
✉ 415–169 Lees Avenue, Ottawa, Ontario, K1S 5M2
☎ 613-565-7660
🖥 www.prostatitis.org/canada

Heart and Stroke Foundation of Canada
✉ 222 Queen Street, Suite 1402, Ottawa, Ontario, K1P 5V9
☎ 613-569-4361
🖥 www.heartandstroke.ca

Prostate Cancer Research Foundation of Canada
✉ 1262 Don Mills Road, Suite 1-F, Toronto, Ontario, M3B 2W7
☎ 1-888-255-0333
🖥 www.prostatecancer.on.ca

Further reading

Susan Aldridge, *Hair Loss: The Answers* (Self-help Direct; London, 1997)

Ian Banks, *Ask Dr Ian about Men's Health* (The Blackstaff Press; Belfast, 1997)

Helen Beare and Neil Priddy, *The Cancer Guide for Men* (Sheldon Press; London, 1999)

Stefan Bechtel and Laurence Roy Stains, *Sex: A Man's Guide* (Rodale Press; Emmaus, PA, 1996)

Nikki Bradford, *Men's Health Matters: The Complete A–Z of Male Health* (Vermilion; London, 1995)

Sarah Brewer, *The Complete Book of Men's Health* (Thorsons; London, 1995)

Steve Carroll, *The Which? Guide to Men's Health* (Which?; London, 1999)

Mick Cooper and Peter Baker, *The MANual: The Complete Man's Guide to Life* (Thorsons; London, 1996)

The Diagram Group, *Man's Body: An Owner's Manual* (Wordsworth Editions; Ware, Herts, 1998)

John Diamond, *C: Because Cowards Get Cancer Too ...* (Vermilion; London, 1999)

Garry Egger, *Trim For Life: 201 Tips for Effective Weight Control* (Allen & Unwin; St Leonards, Australia, 1997)

Oliver Gillie, *Regaining Potency: The Answer to Male Impotence* (Self-help Direct; London, 1997)

Daniel Goleman, *Emotional Intelligence: Why it Can Matter More Than IQ* (Bloomsbury; London, 1996)

Keith Hopcroft and Alistair Moulds, *A Bloke's Diagnose It Yourself Guide to Health* (Oxford University Press; Oxford, 2000)

Charles B. Inlander, et al., *Men's Health and Wellness Encyclopedia* (Macmillan; New York, 1998)

Michael Korda, *Man to Man: Surviving Prostate Cancer* (Warner Books; London, 1998)

Paul Martin, *The Sickening Mind: Brain, Behaviour, Immunity and Disease* (Flamingo; London, 1997)

Dean Ornish, *Love and Survival: The Scientific Basis for the Healing Power of Intimacy* (HarperCollins; New York, 1998)

Jim Pollard, *All Right, Mate? An Easy Intro to Men's Health* (Vista; London, 1999)

Terrence Real, *I Don't Want to Talk About It: Overcoming the Secret Legacy of Male Depression* (Fireside; New York, 1998)

Christopher Reeve, *Still Me* (Arrow; London, 1999)

Lee Rodwell, *You and Your Prostate* (Self-help Direct; London, 1997)

Jonathon Savill and Richard Smedley, *No More Mr Fat Guy: The Nutrition and Fitness Programme for Men!* (Vermilion; London, 1998)

Peter Shalit, *Living Well: The Gay Man's Essential Health Guide* (Alyson; Los Angeles, 1998)

INDEX